RADICAL HEALING

A Stage 4 Cancer Survivor's Holistic Blueprint
for Recovery and Renewal

THE MEDS METHOD
Meditation • Exercise • Diet • Sleep

BY
PURNA PAREEK

First Edition, 2026
ISBN: 979-8-9950443-7-6 (Paperback)
ISBN: 979-8-9950443-8-3 (Hardback)

Printed in the United States of America

DEDICATION

To every warrior facing a life-threatening diagnosis
Don't give up.
You have the power within you to heal yourself.

And

to my family and friends
who walked every step of this journey with me

IMPORTANT MEDICAL DISCLAIMER

This book is not intended as a substitute for medical advice from physicians. The reader should regularly consult a physician in matters relating to their health and particularly with respect to any symptoms that may require diagnosis or medical attention.

The author is not a physician or licensed healthcare provider. The information in this book represents personal experience and research, not medical advice or clinical recommendations. Every cancer is different, and what worked for one person may not work for another.

Always consult with qualified healthcare professionals before making any changes to your treatment plan. Do not discontinue conventional treatment without discussing with your oncologist.

AUTHOR'S NOTE: TWO JOURNEYS

This book chronicles two parallel journeys that unfolded simultaneously yet revealed themselves at different speeds. The first journey—the physical healing from Stage 4 Glioblastoma—was immediate, urgent, and measurable. The second journey—the spiritual evolution that transformed not just my health but my entire understanding of existence—emerged gradually, like a photograph developing in slow motion.

When I first developed the MEDS Method (Meditation, Exercise, Diet, and Sleep), I approached it as an engineer would: systematically, mechanically, desperately seeking a formula to save my life. What I discovered over time was that this "formula" was merely the doorway to something far more profound—a complete transformation of consciousness that would teach me that healing is not just about surviving, but about awakening to who we truly are.

[Throughout this book, you'll notice these bracketed insights—retrospective understandings that came later, showing how my comprehension evolved over time. They represent the deep wisdom that only comes through lived experience.]

ABOUT THE AUTHOR

Purna Pareek is a Stage 4 Glioblastoma survivor, serial entrepreneur, and the creator of the MEDS Method—a holistic healing framework built on Meditation, Exercise, Diet, and Sleep. Diagnosed with terminal brain cancer in 2019 and given months to live, he declined further conventional treatment and committed fully to natural and integrative healing. Six years later, he is cancer-free.

Before his diagnosis, Purna built and successfully exited three technology companies in Silicon Valley. He served as senior executive in multiple public companies following the acquisitions of his companies. He holds a BS degree in Electrical Engineering from Birla Institute of Technology and a master's in Computer Engineering from Brigham Young University.

Since retiring in 2026, Purna has dedicated himself to writing and advocacy, sharing his story with patients, families, and communities navigating serious illnesses. He lives in the San Francisco Bay Area, California with his wife and children.

Radical Healing is his first book.

Contents

PREFACE

Six years ago, I was diagnosed with brain cancer—a moment that instantly reordered my life. The prognosis was grim, and I was forced to confront not only my mortality, but the deeper question of how I wanted to live whatever time I had left.

In the early days, I approached healing in the most practical way I could. I needed structure, something tangible to hold onto when fear and uncertainty threatened to overwhelm me. That led me to develop a simple framework—what I later came to call the MEDS approach—which helped me take consistent, intentional steps toward recovery.

At first, my focus was on the physical aspects of illness. But as time went on, I began to see that healing could not be confined to the body alone. My mindset, emotional patterns, and inner state played a far greater role than I had initially understood. Gradually, the process expanded to include the whole person—body, mind, and something more subtle, yet deeply influential.

What surprised me most was that as my health improved, an inner shift was taking place as well. Paying close attention to my body led me to listen more carefully to my thoughts, my fears, and eventually to a deeper sense of awareness that had little to do with belief and everything to do with experience. In learning how to heal, I also learned how to listen—to my body, my mind, and to a deeper intelligence that had been present all along. Healing became not just a physical recovery, but a quiet spiritual transformation that unfolded naturally along the way.

Many of my friends were surprised by how I handled the illness. Some admired my determination to explore healing approaches beyond the conventional treatments most commonly recommended. As they watched my progress, they began sharing my story with others—family members, friends, and loved ones facing similar diagnoses. Before long, I found myself in conversations with people searching not only for medical options, but for meaning, agency, and hope.

Cancer touches nearly every American family. Despite enormous investments in research and treatment, many people continue to struggle—not only with the disease itself, but with the physical and emotional toll that often accompanies aggressive interventions. For this reason, more patients are seeking ways to support their healing, sometimes alongside standard care, and sometimes when conventional options are limited or intolerable.

I was one of those people. What I learned through my experience gradually took shape as a framework others asked me to share—a way of approaching healing that was practical, adaptable, and grounded in lived experience. This book is the result of those conversations.

It is not meant to replace medical care or offer guarantees. Rather, it is an invitation to engage with healing as a holistic process—one that honors the body, the mind, and the deeper dimensions of being human. If these insights help even a small number of people approach their journey with greater clarity, courage, and inner alignment, then this book will have served its purpose.

Let me be clear: **I am not a physician**, and I'm not offering medical advice in this book. My credentials are not medical degrees but rather the lived experience of walking through fire and emerging on the other side. What follows is not a protocol. It's a **personal blueprint**, one that may resonate with you, or inspire you to find your own. It's a map drawn from my own terrain, and while your landscape may differ, the fundamental principles of navigation might still apply. My goal is not to tell you what to do, but to offer what helped me, in case it sparks something for you. My deepest hope is that it illuminates possibilities you may not have considered, empowering you to explore your own path to wholeness.

It is in that spirit that I dedicate this book to the thousands of warriors battling this dreadful disease. Don't give up. You have the power within you to heal yourself. Believe that you can, and the Universe will bring together the resources you need to make healing a reality in your life.

Be well!

Throughout this book, I use 'I' to describe my personal journey and 'we' when referring to the moments and decisions my wife and I shared together.

PART *One*

THE DIAGNOSIS

The Journey Begins

CHAPTER 1:
BEFORE AND AFTER

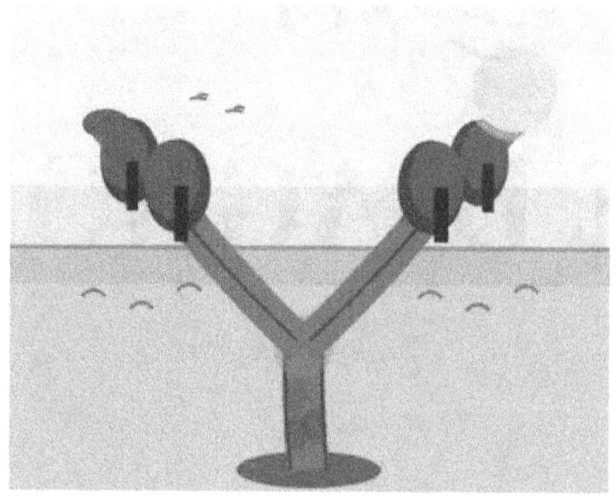

INTRODUCTION

Before this journey began, life felt predictable, comfortable, and steady. I wasn't extraordinary, just a regular person who found joy in simple things. Family dinners, weekend hikes, workouts at the gym, table tennis at the local club, and quiet evenings reading about philosophy and science filled my days with satisfaction and peace. I was grateful for good health and a happy family. As a Silicon Valley startup entrepreneur, I enjoyed technology and building companies with great products.

I never imagined that an ordinary afternoon at the gym would soon split my life into two parts: before and after.

This simple divide, before and after, is how I've come to think of my journey. Not in terms of loss, but in terms of awareness. Life before cancer was lived with a certain momentum, a rhythm built on confidence and consistency. Life after cancer? It was an awakening. An invitation to slow down, look deeper, and live more intentionally.

And the truth is, even in the face of a diagnosis like mine, I never had a breakdown. I didn't collapse under fear or despair. I didn't ask, "Why me?" I've always had spiritual grounding, a naturally optimistic mindset, and a firm belief in the power of resilience. I don't let negative thoughts take root, and that made all the difference.

Some people might find that hard to believe. But if you've lived as an entrepreneur or someone who takes risks, you'll understand. I've faced unknowns before. I've navigated storms. I've always come out the other side stronger. So when cancer came knocking on my door, I looked it in the eye and said, "Let's go."

I knew this journey would test me. I also knew that I would be okay, no matter what the outcome. That deep-seated confidence and optimistic attitude became my armor. It has served me well all my life and gave me space to respond with clarity instead of fear.

LET'S REWIND

It was May 2019, a bright, uneventful day. I wrapped up work at the office and headed to the gym like I usually did. Table tennis was more than a hobby; it was a form of exercise and relaxation for me. The back-and-forth rhythm, the sharp focus, the joy of movement—all of it gave me clarity and presence.

But that day, something was off. My timing was weird. I missed easy shots. My balance felt strange, and I couldn't quite get into the usual flow. I told myself it was just one of those days—low energy, not focusing on the game. Perhaps my vision was getting blurry because of aging. But a small voice in the back of my mind said otherwise.

FOR READERS EXPERIENCING EARLY SYMPTOMS

This is perhaps the most important lesson I can share with you. Our bodies are constantly communicating with us, sending subtle signals long before major symptoms appear. In my case, the tumor was likely growing for months, possibly years, before that day at the table tennis table. Cancer rarely announces itself with a dramatic entrance; it whispers before it shouts.

Looking back, I realize there had been other subtle signs I'd dismissed: occasional mild headaches that I attributed to stress, moments of slight confusion during complex work tasks that I blamed on being tired, and even some minor changes in my sleep patterns. We live such busy lives that we often ignore these gentle warnings, explaining them away with more convenient explanations.

Over the next few days, other strange things happened. I started walking unevenly. My vision would blur unexpectedly. I had difficulty focusing on the screen in front of me, missing a few characters on the left side. Once, while walking through my home, I veered slightly to the left without realizing it. I started running into objects that were far on the left side. Then it began happening frequently.

After several incidents, I realized that while grocery shopping, I often bumped into people or their carts on my left side. On the road, I had a few close calls when a fast-moving car suddenly cut into my lane from the left. Those moments were frightening, because I wasn't aware of the car's presence unless I was fully focused on it.

My wife noticed it too.

THE POWER OF HAVING AN OBSERVER

One crucial advantage I had was my wife's watchful eye. Sometimes the people closest to us notice changes we can't see ourselves. They might observe that we're speaking differently, moving differently, or acting in ways that seem slightly "off" to them, even when we feel normal. If someone you trust mentions they've noticed changes in you, don't dismiss their concerns—they might be seeing something important that you're too close to notice.

These weren't just random slip-ups. Something deeper was going on.

Still, I didn't panic. I'm not the panicking type. My first instinct was to investigate, not react. I decided to book an appointment with my optometrist, thinking that my vision was getting worse and perhaps I needed a new pair of glasses.

SEEKING ANSWERS

The optometrist ran several tests, examined my vision thoroughly, and told me everything seemed normal. There was nothing wrong with my eyes physically. She suggested I see an ophthalmologist.

After running several tests, the ophthalmologist couldn't find anything wrong with the physical structure of my eyes either. She suggested I see a neuro-ophthalmologist who specializes in neurological and brain disorders. But something in her tone suggested she wasn't satisfied with that conclusion. She handed me a referral to a neurologist "just to rule out something more serious."

That phrase, "just to rule out", stuck with me. It was meant to be reassuring, but it had the opposite effect. Neurological issues were out of my comfort zone. This wasn't like managing a project or solving a business challenge. This was my brain. My identity. My life. I made the appointment.

The neurologist listened carefully, took notes, and ordered a brain MRI scan. I went in a few days later, lay down on the table, and listened to the loud rhythmic clicks of the MRI machine's magnets overhead. I didn't feel scared, just focused. I wanted answers. And I was about to get them.

CHAPTER 2:
THE VERDICT

In the middle of difficulty lies opportunity.
— **Albert Einstein**

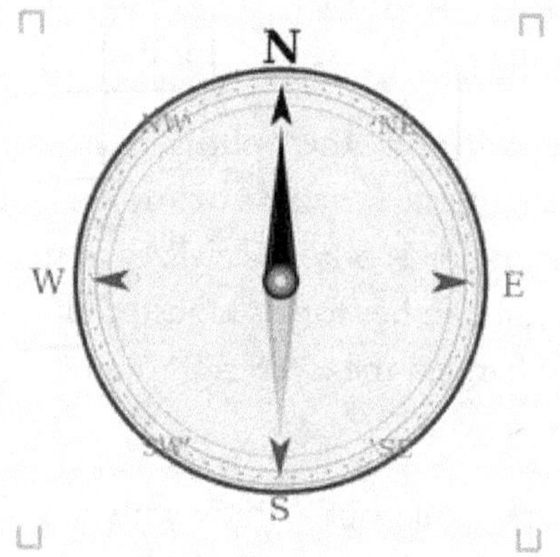

THE MOMENT OF TRUTH

The next day, after the MRI scan results were available, my personal physician called and asked me to come to her office to discuss the findings.

I sat in my doctor's office, waiting. She pulled up the scan results on her screen and turned toward me, her face serious but gentle. My physician was a soft-spoken, young woman. It was probably the first time she had delivered a terminal cancer diagnosis to anyone, so I can only imagine how tense she must have been.

Finally, she turned toward us and delivered the news. "We've found a mass in your brain," she said slowly. "It appears to be a brain tumor. It's called Glioblastoma."

UNDERSTANDING GLIOBLASTOMA

Glioblastoma (GBM) is considered the most aggressive form of brain cancer. It's what's called a "grade 4" tumor, meaning it grows and spreads rapidly. The cells look very abnormal under a microscope and multiply quickly. What makes GBM particularly challenging is that it sends out tiny finger-like projections into healthy brain tissue, making it nearly impossible to remove completely through surgery alone. The median survival time is typically 6-12 months, with only about 5% of patients surviving five years. These are the stark statistics that I would learn in the days to come.

I didn't flinch. I had no immediate reaction. I just listened. Perhaps because I didn't know what it meant. I had never heard the term Glioblastoma or GBM before in my life. The only thing I could immediately realize was that cancer is not good no matter where it is, but it could be serious if it's in the brain. As an always-optimistic person, my thought was: perhaps there's some mistake. Maybe the MRI reading isn't accurate.

In that moment, the world didn't spin out of control. Instead, it felt like everything slowed down. I was watching it all happen from a quiet place inside me.

Okay, I thought. This is happening. We will deal with it.

THE PSYCHOLOGY OF CRISIS RESPONSE

Later, I would learn that my calm reaction isn't uncommon. Psychologists call this "emotional numbing" or "dissociation"—the mind's way of protecting us from overwhelming information. Some people collapse, others get angry, and still others, like me, enter a state of hyper-calm focus. There's no right or wrong way to receive devastating news. Your initial reaction doesn't predict how you'll handle the journey ahead.

It may sound strange, but I felt incredibly calm. I didn't feel like a victim. I felt like a participant in something I couldn't yet define. I knew I was going to have to make big decisions quickly. I also knew that panicking wouldn't serve me. As a founder, I had trained myself to look at crises not as threats, but as problems to be solved. This diagnosis, in that initial moment, felt like the ultimate startup challenge.

My mind didn't go to worst-case scenarios. Instead, I felt that I would come out just fine on the other side. It went to logistics, to clarity, to next steps. That's how I've always lived my life, and cancer wasn't going to change that. I looked at the doctor and asked, "What do we do next?"

She suggested I see a brain surgeon who specializes in Glioblastoma. My local health provider had a brain surgeon on staff. She referred me to him and recommended that I not waste any time because the tumor was almost 4 cm and it was Stage 4 cancer. That means it's terminal cancer, and generally, there is no cure. Most people don't live beyond 6 to 12 months after diagnosis.

As we drove home from the doctor's office, the reality was beginning to hit. The fear of the unknown was beginning to emerge from the background. We went home and sat down at the dining table to plan our next move.

IMMEDIATE THOUGHTS, UNFINISHED BUSINESS

After learning I may have only 6 to 12 months left, I realized there were important matters to address for those who depend on me. My motivation came from taking care of my responsibilities, not from fear. I'm trained to think logically, so I identified three important issues to address:

1. Financial security for the family and loved ones

2. Attending my daughter's wedding that was scheduled in three months

3. Selling my company to relieve myself from day-to-day business operations

While my mind was creating a to-do list, my heart was quietly grappling with the potential goodbyes these tasks represented. Fortunately, as an entrepreneur, I had done well and felt financially secure. That assured me that my wife and children would have enough to live their lives even if I wasn't around as the primary breadwinner. This was a great relief.

My two children were grown adults working full-time in the high-tech industry. They were settled in their jobs and careers. They didn't need my help anymore.

My daughter was getting married, and her wedding was scheduled for September, four months after my diagnosis. Since this was within the six-month timeframe, I felt happy that I would be able to attend her wedding. Another box checked.

A few months before the cancer diagnosis, we were in serious conversations with a company in an adjacent business that wanted to acquire my business. We were in a due diligence process before the diagnosis. My cancer diagnosis would definitely derail the deal, I thought. No one would want to buy a startup company whose founder isn't expected to live very long. I needed to deal with this issue.

RESEARCH AND LEARNING PHASE

We decided to learn everything we could about cancer, especially Glioblastoma (GBM), to truly understand what we were facing. My wife, an avid reader, immediately put our family's collective research skills to work, scouring the internet for articles, books, and scientific publications on GBM. We watched YouTube videos on cancer biology and how people were dealing with it.

The information overload - and how to navigate it: In the age of the internet, cancer patients face a unique challenge: too much information, much of it contradictory or outdated. We found ourselves drowning in statistics, treatment protocols, clinical trials, and survivor stories. Some sources were hopeful, others terrifying. My advice to anyone facing a similar diagnosis: start with reputable medical institutions (Mayo Clinic, Johns Hopkins, National Cancer Institute) for basic facts, then dive deeper into specific treatment centers. Avoid online forums initially; they can be helpful later, but early on, they often increase anxiety rather than provide clarity.

We also learned to distinguish between different types of information. Statistical data helped us understand the general landscape, but individual stories reminded us that statistics don't determine personal outcomes. We were looking for two things: the best medical care available, and examples of people who had exceeded expectations.

FINDING THE RIGHT SURGEON

Our priority, however, was to find the best possible brain surgeon for the operation. We compiled a list of the top hospitals in the U.S. specializing in GBM surgery: Stanford, UCSF, Mayo Clinic, Cleveland Clinic, and Duke. My wife wasted no time contacting each one to determine how quickly we could get an appointment. We went on scouring the internet and YouTube videos for any information we could find on GBM and read the comments on forums about other people's experiences. One forum would be filled with stories of miraculous recoveries from a specific diet, while another would vehemently debunk it. The emotional whiplash was exhausting.

The importance of speed vs. the right choice: One thing we learned quickly is that with GBM, time matters, but the right surgeon matters more. A tumor growing at this rate needed attention within weeks, not months, but rushing into surgery with the wrong team could be catastrophic. We had to balance urgency with thoroughness in our research.

My primary physician referred me to a GBM surgeon at our local hospital. As we began to grasp how serious this diagnosis was, it no longer felt right to simply place my trust in a local brain surgeon. This was the moment to dig deeper, to rigorously research the surgeon's credentials, because I was about to entrust my brain—and my life—to a very serious operation.

Since Stanford is nearby, my wife managed to secure an appointment with a surgeon there within the same week. At the same time, we discovered that UCSF boasts some of the nation's leading brain cancer surgeons, though their schedules are notoriously full. Undeterred, she called the UCSF Cancer Center. The nurse who answered was kind but explained they were fully booked, except for a last-minute cancellation that had just occurred. If we could arrive within the hour, she could fit us in. We seized the opportunity and made the hour-long drive to UCSF in San Francisco.

There, Dr. Theodosopoulos, an accomplished surgeon with over 2,000 GBM surgeries to his name, reviewed my MRI and confirmed it was a Stage 4 brain tumor requiring immediate intervention. He assured us that he had seen enough cases like mine and made us feel very comfortable that he was a highly qualified surgeon I could trust. He said he could clear his schedule to operate that week since it was an urgent case. Before surgery, a more detailed MRI was needed to accurately map my brain and determine the precise entry point.

Dr. Theodosopoulos explained the procedure: he would need to open my skull with a saw to access the right occipital lobe, where the tumor had taken hold. The occipital lobe controls vision, which explained my impaired sight on the left side. After removing the tumor, he would close the skull with surgical staples, much like a heavy-duty office stapler. Healing would take about three weeks, after which the staples would be removed. I was struck by how basic this aspect of brain surgery remains.

Despite my apprehensions, Dr. Theodosopoulos's confidence and expertise reassured us. He took time to walk us through every detail, and by the end of our meeting, we felt so comfortable that I asked my wife to cancel our Stanford appointment scheduled a couple of hours later. We felt certain we had found the right surgeon.

With the surgery scheduled, the wheels were finally in motion. The universe seemed to cooperate to bring us the best surgeon in the fastest possible timeframe. We were relieved.

The next step was to communicate with my children and share the difficult news.

FAMILY STRENGTH AND UNITY

Telling my family was harder than hearing the diagnosis. I wasn't afraid of their reaction; I just didn't want them to suffer. But I also knew I couldn't go through this alone.

That night, we called our children. We gathered around the dining table and shared the diagnosis. I told them that I had Stage 4 brain cancer. It was a terminal illness. Most patients don't survive for more than 6 to 12 months. The survival rate is less than 5%. So we needed to prepare ourselves for the possibility that I might not be around for too long.

The air in the room seemed to pause. I saw the shock in their eyes. Then, without a word, we hugged. All of us. There were tears, silent, strong, human emotions.

We stood in a circle, holding one another. It was the first time I'd seen my kids cry like that. But even through their tears, they showed courage. One of them said, "We're with you, Dad. Whatever it takes."

Later that evening, I told them I wanted to give them access to all my financial accounts and important documents, not out of fear, but out of responsibility. If anything happened, I wanted them to be prepared. My wife and I sat with folders and spreadsheets, organizing everything. It gave me a sense of order in chaos.

After dinner, we did something simple but powerful: we played music, a collection of 70s and 80s songs that even my kids had begun to like.

Then the playlist started playing "Dust in the Wind" by Kansas. This is one of my favorite songs from my teenage years, but that day it took on a different meaning altogether and hit me hard. It portrayed the mortality and fragility of life. The lyrics were so relevant to my situation.

I close my eyes, only for a moment, and the moment's gone. All my dreams pass before my eyes like curiosity. Dust in the wind, all we are is dust in the wind.

Same old song, just a drop of water in the endless sea, All we do, crumble to the ground though we refuse to see, Dust in the wind, All we are is dust in the wind.

Don't hang on, nothing lasts forever but the earth and sky It's still far away, And all your money wouldn't another minute buy Everything is dust in the wind.

I listened in silence. The song wasn't sad, but grounding, bringing tears to my eyes — and it still does. It reminded me of life's impermanence and the importance of living fully and loving deeply while we can.

My wife sat beside me as I explained to our children everything we had just learned. She didn't say a word at first. She simply reached out and held my hand. Then, quietly, with tears forming, she said, "We'll face this together."

That moment bonded us as a family. It gave us emotional clarity. From that point forward, we weren't navigating cancer; we were navigating life together.

CHAPTER 3:
INTO THE FIRE

The cave you fear to enter holds the treasure you seek.
— Joseph Campbell

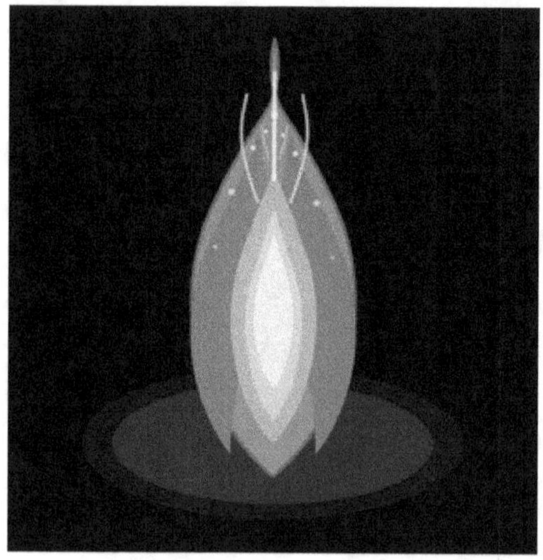

THE SURGERY

Everything moved quickly after that. I was scheduled for surgery within days.

The night before, I lay in my bed, looking at the ceiling, my mind surprisingly calm. I thought about my kids, my wife, and the people I loved. I thought about all the things I had yet to experience, and how grateful I was for what I already had.

I wasn't afraid of dying. I accepted the possible outcome. Now I was curious about living.

The next morning, we checked into the hospital. The surgical team introduced themselves, confident, focused professionals. Their calm demeanor reassured me. After going through a few hours of pre-surgical procedures, I said goodbye to my wife and kids and was taken to the operating room. I remember the cold feeling of the operating room, the bright lights above.

The doctor explained the procedure and put the oxygen mask on my face. I heard the gentle voice of the anesthesiologist saying, "We'll take good care of you." Lying on the operating table, I took a deep breath and decided to go into a meditation state. In a few moments, darkness fell and I lost consciousness. I was in the void under anesthesia.

When I woke up, there was a strange awareness. My thoughts were cloudy, but I was still me. I recognized the doctor's voice. I moved my fingers, then my toes.

Relief washed over me. The nurse moved me from the operating room to the recovery room where my wife and kids were waiting for me. They hugged me and said the surgery had gone well.

Later, the surgeon came to the room and told me they had removed most of the tumor. There would be a long recovery process. Some risks remained. But overall, the operation had gone well.

I was deeply grateful, not just to the doctors, but to life itself.

AFTER SURGERY

The brain is the most delicate organ in the body, weighing just about two pounds yet responsible for controlling every bodily function. During surgery, the surgeon must exercise extreme caution to avoid disturbing or damaging any other areas, as even a slight misstep could result in the loss of speech, language, or movement abilities. After my operation, the surgeon visited my room to check on me. Remarkably, despite having undergone such a complex procedure, I felt completely normal. I even wondered why everyone seemed so concerned. Little did I realize what challenges still lay ahead.

Soon after, a nurse encouraged me to get up and walk with her close to the wall. This was to ensure my motor skills were intact. The only lingering issue was the impaired vision in my left eye, which remained unchanged. The surgeon had removed the part of my brain responsible for processing signals from that eye because the tumor had overtaken those cells. Now, with that section gone, there was simply nothing left to interpret the optical signals, even though my eye and optic nerve themselves were still functioning. Specifically, the part of my right occipital lobe that managed left-eye vision had been surgically removed, resulting in the loss of most of my peripheral vision on that side. That was where the cancer had formed its tumor. The surgery successfully removed the colony of malignant cells.

Aside from this, I felt surprisingly well. I soon met with my oncologist, who would oversee the next stage of my care. I was relieved to learn that there were no restrictions on my diet or lifestyle; my only instructions were to go home, rest, recover, and return after three weeks.

Brain surgery involves opening the skull to reach the affected area. It's a surprisingly mechanical process: the surgeons use a saw to cut open the skull, and after the procedure, they close the opening with surgical staples. Once the incision has healed, the staples are removed.

Three weeks after the surgery, I returned to the hospital. The medical team examined my skull, determined that the incision had healed well, and safely removed the staples.

MANAGING WORK DURING TREATMENT

Given the seriousness of my diagnosis, I decided to keep it strictly confidential, telling only family and close friends. At work, I kept things intentionally vague—mentioning only that I was dealing with some health issues requiring treatment. I understood that revealing a terminal diagnosis would destabilize the business, creating the kind of uncertainty I was determined to prevent.

Post-surgery, my altered appearance posed a challenge. The visible changes to my skull meant I wore a cap constantly, hiding the scars and stitches from view. This required careful navigation with my team—acknowledging that something was happening while maintaining firm boundaries about the details. I had to strike a balance between transparency about my changed appearance and protecting both the company's stability and my personal privacy.

The three-week recovery period following surgery was dedicated to rest, healing, and building strength for the upcoming chemotherapy and radiation. At the end of those three weeks, the nurse removed the stitches and allowed the wound to heal naturally. I couldn't help but notice the irony—the staples holding my skull together were remarkably similar to ordinary office staples. For all the complexity of brain surgery, this particular aspect felt surprisingly mechanical, almost mundane.

POST-SURGERY, RADIATION TREATMENT

After surgery came radiation, five days a week, for six weeks. They molded a custom mask that locked my head in place, bolting it to the table. It was painless physically, but emotionally challenging.

The reality of radiation therapy: What they don't tell you about radiation is how profoundly isolating it can feel. You're strapped to a table, completely alone in a room, while invisible rays penetrate your skull and body. The machine makes sounds like a science fiction movie, whirring, clicking, buzzing. The technicians leave the room and speak to you through an intercom. Each session lasted about 45 minutes, but it felt like hours.

The worst part wasn't the physical discomfort; it was the psychological weight of knowing that these X-rays, while targeting cancer cells, were also damaging healthy brain tissue. Every session was a calculated gamble: kill more cancer than healthy cells, and hope the balance tips in your favor.

Lying still while the machine buzzed around my skull made time feel surreal. I focused on my breathing like I was in meditation, trying to be as calm as possible. The doctor had instructed me to be as still as possible so they could target the area where the tumor was and kill as many remaining cancer cells as possible. I mentally visualized how the X-rays were zapping the cancer cells in the tumor.

Visualization as a coping tool: During each session, I developed a detailed visualization practice. I imagined the radiation as precise light sabers, cutting through malignant cells while leaving healthy tissue intact. I pictured my immune system as an army of warriors, cleaning up the battlefield after each session. This wasn't just positive thinking; it gave me something active to do during those long, helpless minutes. Later, I learned that many cancer patients develop similar mental practices, and some research suggests that positive visualization may actually support healing by reducing stress hormones that can suppress immune function.

I began taking Temozolomide, a chemotherapy pill that damages cancer cell DNA and can cross the blood-brain barrier, making it effective against brain tumors. However, radiation also harms healthy brain cells, which is an unavoidable trade-off, much like losing your own soldiers in battle alongside the enemy.

Understanding the side effects, what to expect: The side effects weren't immediate, which was almost worse than if they had been. For the first week, I felt fine and began to think maybe I'd be one of the lucky ones who tolerated treatment well. I congratulated myself on how well I was handling the first week. I was going to the office every day and pretending that I was perfectly normal. I didn't tell anyone in the office about the diagnosis. Then, gradually, the effects accumulated. Fatigue that felt different from anything I'd experienced, not like being tired after a workout, but like my cellular energy was being drained. Brain fog that made simple decisions feel overwhelming. Food began to taste metallic, and even my favorite meals became unappealing.

The side effects of this therapy were relentless. Fatigue. Brain fog. Nausea. Metallic taste. Weight loss. It felt like I was disappearing from the inside out.

The initial three weeks were manageable. I was able to cope with the challenges during this period. Chemotherapy pills taken at night resulted in vomiting and made sleep difficult. The treatment regimen included radiation therapy in the morning and chemotherapy at night, placing significant physical strain on the entire body.

The sleep crisis, and why it matters so much: What I didn't understand initially was how crucial sleep would be to my recovery. Sleep isn't just rest; it's when your body does its most important healing work. During deep sleep, your brain cleans out toxins, your immune system rebuilds, and damaged cells repair themselves. The chemotherapy was not only making me sick but also destroying the very process my body needed most to fight the cancer.

This created a vicious cycle: the treatment made me too sick to sleep well, and the lack of sleep made me less able to tolerate the treatment and fight the disease. Breaking this cycle became one of the most important aspects of my healing journey.

But I kept going.

My wife prepared meals for me, though I wasn't always able to eat them. My children sent messages like "Love you, Dad."

I decided to share the news only with close family members and a few friends. Support from them played an important role during this period. Messages and positive feedback regarding my response to the situation contributed to my motivation to recover.

My objective extended beyond completing treatment; I was also committed to achieving full recovery. Rather than accepting the statistical probabilities of survival at face value, I recognized that exceptions exist, and I was determined to be among them.

We began researching nutritional therapies, functional medicine, and holistic health approaches. I also incorporated short periods of meditation each day, with the intention of self-reflection rather than avoidance.

The experience involved both medical and personal elements.

THE DAILY REALITY OF TREATMENT

Just as I was beginning to stabilize and recover from the brain surgery and stress of treatment, something else started happening.

I had to take chemo pills at night. They had devastating effects. I was throwing up continuously. This was not only uncomfortable, but it completely disturbed my sleep. I didn't know it then, but learning to reclaim my sleep would become one of the most important battles I would fight and win. For all practical purposes, I wasn't getting any sleep at night. Later, I learned that while you sleep, your body repairs tissues, builds muscle, and releases growth hormones. This is vital for recovery from illness, daily wear and tear, and for a strong immune system that fights cancer cells.

My body was being attacked from all sides, chemo and radiation were killing both the cancer cells as well as healthy cells at the same time while the regeneration process was impaired.

EXPLORING CANNABIS-BASED SYMPTOM MANAGEMENT

Through our research, we discovered that CBD and THC combinations had shown promise in helping cancer patients manage treatment side effects, particularly the nausea, vomiting, and pain associated with chemotherapy. Since sleep had become elusive for me, I decided to try a CBD-THC combination that ultimately improved my rest. The side effects were minimal—mainly drowsiness from the THC component. Finding the right dosage required some experimentation to avoid being completely sedated while still achieving the therapeutic benefits. The field continues to evolve, with ongoing research investigating how cannabinoids might support cancer patients beyond just symptom relief.

I was waking up multiple times each night. I couldn't sleep for more than an hour or two at a stretch. I had symptoms of nocturia before the surgery. The doctor prescribed medicine to control frequent urination. Given that this is not an uncommon problem in older adults, I did not pay much attention to it. However, following chemotherapy and radiation therapy, the symptoms worsened.

At first, I attributed it to chemo side effects. But something didn't sit right.

PART *Two*

THE STORM INTENSIFIES

When Challenges Compound

CHAPTER 4:
THE SECOND CANCER

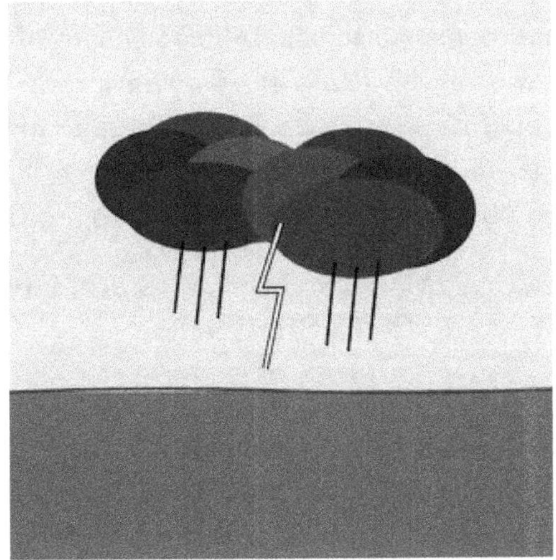

My oncologist suggested that I consult a urologist at UCSF. Given that I was going through brain cancer treatment, she immediately ordered some tests and inspected the inside of the bladder using a camera. Then came the news:

"You have bladder cancer."

They weren't sure if it had infiltrated the bladder wall. If it had, it would be Stage 4 Muscle Invasive cancer. That means it would metastasize and could spread to lymph nodes and ultimately all over the body. This was a very scary scenario. For GBM, we knew that although it's the most aggressive form of cancer, it remains in the brain only. But Stage

4 bladder cancer could spread everywhere quickly once it gets into the bloodstream.

A second, unrelated diagnosis. It had nothing to do with brain cancer.

I paused. I took a deep breath.

This, too? Really?

A STRANGE CALM

When I got yet another scary diagnosis, I didn't feel the fear I thought I would. Instead, a strange calm washed over me. It was like everything I'd already been through had actually prepared me for this. I knew how to react, and it wasn't with panic. It was with a clear head, a strong spirit, and the hopeful outlook I'd fought so hard to maintain. A deep feeling rose up inside me: I'm going to get through this. The ancient wisdom tradition phrase echoed in my head: This too shall pass.

BRAIN AND BLADDER CANCERS: AN UNLIKELY COINCIDENCE

My first fear was metastasis—that the brain tumor had somehow spread to my bladder. But my doctors quickly clarified that this was virtually impossible. The brain exists in its own protected environment, separated from the rest of the body by the blood-brain barrier, which prevents brain cancer cells from infiltrating other organs. These two cancers were entirely unrelated, a medical mystery of sorts.

My oncologists confirmed they were dealing with two independent malignancies. In a strange way, this was supposed to be good news—at least the cancer wasn't spreading systemically. But that consolation was fleeting. Having two separate primary cancers felt less like relief and more like being struck by lightning twice.

THE NIGHTMARE RETURNS, A BIG CHOICE

The plan for my bladder cancer felt like a terrible dream coming true again: more surgery, more chemo, more radiation. I was just barely recovering from six weeks of intense treatment for my brain tumor

(GBM). My body was completely worn out, filled with powerful medicines. The doctors wanted me to take a break, to let my body heal a bit before the next big battle.

But that break became a huge turning point. I had a big choice to make, one that was about much more than just medical procedures. It was about life itself. Surgery and modern medicine had helped me so far, but the quality of that life was slipping away. I saw a never-ending future of radiation and chemo, a life sentence of constant treatment for diseases they said couldn't be cured.

I'd witnessed this happen to a few people I knew. One of them was my business partner's wife. She was diagnosed with GBM, very similar to my case. None of them survived despite multiple surgeries and strong medical intervention. Conventional GBM treatment is often insufficient. It appeared to be a stopgap measure to extend life a bit more.

CHAPTER 5:
THE CROSSROADS

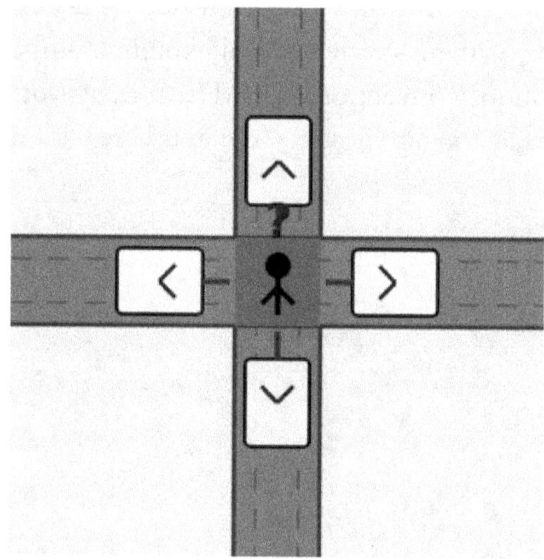

IS SURVIVING THE SAME AS HEALING?

I started to wonder: What if just staying alive wasn't the same as truly healing?

The more I read and learned, the more I felt that real healing was about the whole person, mind, body, and spirit all working together. My main focus and goal began to change significantly. I didn't just want to attack tumors; I wanted to build a strong shield of wellness from the inside. I wanted to create an environment inside my body where sickness just couldn't grow. This was the real start of my transformation, a journey toward a completely different way of living.

THE TERRAIN THEORY VS. GERM THEORY

During my research, I discovered a fundamental philosophical divide in how we think about disease. Traditional Western medicine operates primarily on "germ theory", the idea that disease is caused by external pathogens (germs, toxins, genetic mutations) that invade and attack the body. The solution is to kill the invaders with powerful weapons: chemotherapy, radiation, antibiotics.

But there's another perspective called "terrain theory," which suggests that disease thrives in certain internal environments and cannot take hold in others. Just as mosquitoes breed in stagnant water but not in flowing streams, cancer may flourish in bodies that are stressed, inflamed, nutrient-depleted, and toxic, but struggle to survive in bodies that are alkaline, well-nourished, well-rested, and emotionally balanced.

Both perspectives have merit, but I realized that mainstream medicine focuses almost exclusively on killing the cancer while largely ignoring the terrain that allowed it to grow in the first place. What if I could do both, use medical treatment to remove the immediate threat while simultaneously transforming my internal environment to make it inhospitable to future disease?

I began to understand that modern medicine, even with all its power, was mostly set up to handle symptoms. It couldn't cure my illness, but its side effects were so harsh that it felt like part of me was dying along with the cancer. I faced a tough, almost painful choice: live a longer life but feel half-dead, weak, and constantly sick with new problems, or try other ways of healing that promised dignity and a better quality of life, even if they couldn't promise a full cure.

This book details that journey and the holistic healing blueprint, focused on Mind, Emotions, Diet, and Spirit, that became my guide back to wholeness.

QUALITY OF LIFE VS. QUANTITY OF LIFE

This became the central question of my journey. Medical oncology excels at extending life, adding months or even years to survival statistics. But what kind of life? I met other patients in the treatment center who had been fighting their cancer for years, cycling through different chemotherapy regimens, managing endless side effects, living from scan to scan in a state of chronic anxiety.

I began to realize that for me, six months of feeling truly alive and vibrant might be more valuable than two years of feeling sick and diminished. This wasn't about giving up; it was about redefining what it meant to win the fight against cancer. Winning was no longer about seeing a clean scan in two years; it was about truly tasting my food today, feeling the warmth of the sun on my skin, and being fully present for my daughter's wedding.

In the end, I made a clear and strong choice, to live fully, with purpose, for every day I'm alive. Longevity became a secondary objective.

CHAPTER 6:
TAKING THE LEAP

And the day came when the risk to remain tight in a bud was more painful than the risk it took to blossom.

— **Anaïs Nin**

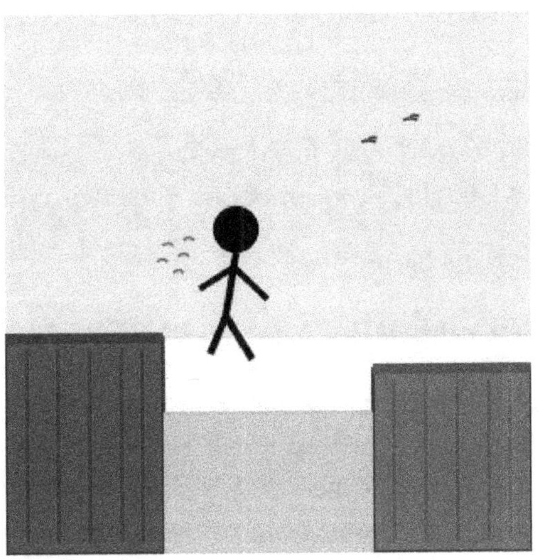

TAKING CHARGE OF MY OWN HEALTH

This choice wasn't about saying no to the medicine that had helped me so far. Instead, it was about adding more tools to my healing kit. I eagerly dove into subjects I'd only glanced at before, meditation, different ways of thinking about life and mind over matter, how the brain works, and how our bodies function. Most importantly, I started to truly listen to my body. It wasn't just a collection of problems anymore, but a wise friend gently sending messages to me.

I came to believe in something important: healing isn't just about not being sick. It's about actively supporting your body's own ability to get well. It became my mission to feed my immune system in every way, so it could fight hard for me. This meant really looking at what I ate, making sure I got deep, restful sleep, and dealing with my stress and emotions.

More than anything, this journey became about taking full responsibility for my own health. I wasn't just a patient anymore, waiting for things to happen to me. I became an active participant in my own well-being, turning my body into a kind of laboratory for my own experiments to discover hopeful and courageous ways to heal.

EMBRACING A HOLISTIC LIFE

That shift in mindset changed everything.

My wife and I chose to make lifestyle changes focused on healing. We reviewed our food, habits, sleep, emotions, and environment.

We started with the basics.

A COMPLETE DIETARY TRANSFORMATION

We transformed our kitchen from the ground up, clearing out processed foods, refined sugars, and anything known to trigger inflammation. This wasn't easy for me—I've always craved something sweet after meals, that satisfying end note to every dish. But learning that cancer cells feed on glucose changed everything. Those beloved desserts had to go.

In their place came a new way of eating: abundant plant-based dishes, nourishing healthy fats, fresh organic ingredients, and mindful hydration throughout the day. We stopped seeing food as mere fuel or comfort and started treating it as our frontline defense—turning every meal into an opportunity for healing.

But this wasn't just about eating "healthy" foods; it was about understanding food as information. Every bite was either feeding cancer or fighting it. Sugar, for example, literally feeds cancer cells, which consume glucose at much higher rates than normal cells. Processed foods create inflammation, which cancer uses to spread. Pesticides and artificial additives burden the liver, which needs to be free to process toxins and support immune function.

I learned about specific anti-cancer foods: cruciferous vegetables like broccoli and cauliflower that contain compounds which help the body eliminate toxins; turmeric and ginger for their powerful anti-inflammatory properties; green tea for its antioxidants; and healthy fats like those found in avocados and wild-caught fish that support brain health and reduce inflammation.

MOVEMENT AS MEDICINE

I also turned to movement, not as punishment or exercise, but as a celebration of life. Walks in nature. Gentle stretching. Breathing deeply while standing barefoot in the garden.

Exercise had always been part of my life, but now I understood it differently. Physical activity doesn't just build muscles, it literally changes the internal environment of your body. It oxygenates tissues, stimulates lymphatic drainage (your body's waste removal system), triggers the release of endorphins and other healing chemicals, and has been shown in studies to directly inhibit tumor growth.

But during treatment, intense exercise was impossible. Instead, we focused on gentle movement that honored where my body was. Some days it was a slow walk around the block. Other days it was simple stretching in bed. The goal wasn't fitness, it was circulation, oxygenation, and maintaining the connection between my mind and body.

SLEEP AS SACRED MEDICINE

Sleep became sacred. I stopped treating rest as an afterthought. Instead, it became a core pillar of my healing strategy. No screens before bed. Calming teas. Guided sleep meditations.

I learned that sleep isn't just recovery time, it's when your immune system does its most important work. During deep sleep, your body produces the most white blood cells, which are your cancer-fighting army. Sleep also triggers the release of melatonin, a powerful antioxidant that has been shown to inhibit tumor growth. Poor sleep, on the other hand, elevates cortisol and other stress hormones that suppress immune function and create inflammation.

We restructured our bedroom into a true sleep sanctuary—dark, cool, and free of screens—and built a consistent nightly routine to signal to my body that it was time to rest and heal. (See Chapter 14 for the full sleep protocol.)

THE SCIENCE OF MEDITATION AND HEALING

And then, there was stillness. Meditation moved from something I "should do" to something I needed. Some days it was just 15 minutes of breath awareness. Other days it was an hour or two, deeper, even transcendental.

What I discovered about meditation surprised me. It's not just relaxation, it's a powerful medical intervention. Studies have shown that regular meditation can measurably boost immune function, reduce inflammation, lower stress hormones, and even influence gene expression in ways that support healing.

But beyond the science, meditation gave me something even more valuable: the ability to be present with my experience without being overwhelmed by it. It taught me to observe thoughts and emotions without being controlled by them. When fear arose, I could acknowledge it without letting it drive my decisions. When pain appeared, I could breathe with it rather than fight against it.

There were no rigid rules, just rhythms. We created healing rituals. Morning gratitude. Evening reflection. Time to simply be.

My wife was my partner in all of this. She made it possible. Her belief in my healing often exceeded my own. Her dedication gave me strength. She wasn't just helping me survive; she was helping me transform.

Healing became our way of life. It was no longer about the fight. It was about the flow.

MOMENTS THAT MATTERED MOST

The real gift of this transformation wasn't just better lab results or improved energy, though those came in time. The real gift was presence.

I began to live in the now. Not in fear of recurrence or the weight of the past, but in the beauty of what was right in front of me.

One moment that stood out was my daughter's wedding.

Just four months after my diagnosis and treatment, I walked her down the aisle and watched her take her vows, fully present. The sun was setting, soft music was playing, and I looked at her with pride, gratitude, and awe. I didn't think about my illness. I didn't think about tomorrow. I was grateful to life that I was alive and well, witnessing this moment.

I held her hand. I smiled for photos. We hugged each other, with more joy than I thought I could feel. That day wasn't about survival. It was about celebration. It was a reminder of what I was truly healing for.

Not just years on the clock, but memories in the heart.

These are the moments cancer can't take away. These are the reasons I chose to live differently. These are the reasons I'll never go back to the way things were.

WHAT CANCER TAUGHT ME ABOUT LIFE

Cancer, oddly enough, became one of my greatest teachers.

It stripped away the noise. The unnecessary. The superficial. It reminded me how much time I had spent rushing through life, checking off boxes, meeting expectations, and postponing joy for "later."

It taught me that later is not guaranteed.

THE GIFT OF FORCED PRESENCE

Before cancer, I thought I was living intentionally. But I often found myself caught in autopilot, doing things because they were expected, working hard to excel at work, not because they were essential. Cancer pulled the emergency brake. It forced me to ask: What truly matters?

Suddenly, the urgent became irrelevant, and the important became obvious. Closing that next business deal? Not important. Spending time with my family? Essential. Worrying about financial projections? Meaningless. Watching a sunset on the beach in silence? Profound.

Cancer gave me what I call "mortality clarity", the sharp focus that comes from knowing that time is limited. This clarity isn't available to most people until they face their own mortality, but it's one of life's greatest gifts. It cuts through all the noise and reveals what actually matters.

I learned that it's not about chasing more. It's about savoring what's already here now.

EMOTIONAL HEALING AS PART OF PHYSICAL HEALING

I learned that healing doesn't just happen in the body, it happens in the soul. In the quiet acceptance of what is. In the courage to feel deeply. In the decision to choose peace, even when circumstances suggest otherwise.

I learned that emotions are part of healing. I allowed myself to grieve and feel pain, not just because of the diagnosis, but the illusion of control. I allowed myself to feel fear, but I didn't let it run the show. I allowed joy to reenter my life, not as a reward, but as a necessity.

One of the most powerful discoveries was that unprocessed emotions create physical tension and inflammation in the body. Chronic stress, anger, resentment, and fear literally suppress immune function and create an environment where disease can thrive. Healing required me to not just change what I ate or how I slept, but to examine and release emotional patterns that had been affecting my health for years.

THE INTERCONNECTED WEB OF WELLNESS

I also saw how everything interconnects, mind, body, spirit, relationships, environment. They're not separate systems. They're one interconnected ecosystem. When one part heals, the others follow.

This was perhaps the most important insight of my entire journey. Western medicine tends to compartmentalize, the neurologist focuses on the brain, the oncologist on cancer cells, the cardiologist on the heart. But the body doesn't operate in compartments. Everything affects everything else.

My stress levels affected my sleep quality. My sleep quality affected my immune function. My immune function affected my body's ability to fight cancer. My diet affected my energy levels. My energy levels affected my mood. My mood affected my relationships. My relationships affected my stress levels. It was all connected.

LIVING WITH URGENCY VS. LIVING WITH ANXIETY

I have had a lot of worries in my life, most of which never happened. —Mark Twain

Cancer taught me the difference between urgency and anxiety. Anxiety is about feared futures that may never come. Urgency is about making the most of the present moment. Anxiety depletes energy and creates stress. Urgency creates focus and motivation.

I learned to live with urgency, to prioritize what mattered, to have important conversations, to experience beauty deeply, to love without reservation. But I also learned to release anxiety about outcomes I couldn't control. I couldn't control whether the cancer would return, but I could control how fully I lived each day I was given.

And maybe the most important lesson: You don't need to wait for a crisis to wake up.

MY INVITATION TO YOU

If you're reading this, you or someone dear to you might be at the beginning of a journey. Or maybe you're somewhere in the messy middle. Wherever you are, I want you to know this:

You are not powerless.

You don't have to accept fear as your baseline. You don't have to surrender your agency. You can choose to be a participant in your healing. You can choose how you show up each day, what you nourish yourself with physically, emotionally, and spiritually.

A FRAMEWORK, NOT A FORMULA

This book is not a medical guide. It's a healing blueprint. A personal one. I'll share everything that helped me, from the mindset shifts to the dietary changes, from the breathwork to the deep meditation. I'll talk about supplements, rest, science, spirituality, and everything in between.

But none of this is about copying what I did. It's about creating a framework that you can make your own. Healing isn't linear. It isn't one-size-fits-all. It's personal. It's alive.

THE JOURNEY AHEAD

In the chapters that follow, we'll explore each aspect of holistic healing in detail. You'll learn about the specific nutritional protocols that became my daily medicine, the meditation practices that shifted my internal state, the sleep optimization techniques that supercharged my recovery, and the emotional healing work that addressed root causes I never knew existed.

I'll share the science behind why these approaches work, but more importantly, I'll show you how to adapt them to your unique situation. Whether you're dealing with cancer, another serious illness, or simply want to optimize your health and prevent disease, these principles apply.

I will also address the practical challenges: how to work with your medical team while pursuing integrative approaches, how to navigate the information overload, how to maintain hope without falling into denial, and how to build a support system that honors your choices.

THREE KEY PRINCIPLES TO REMEMBER

As we begin this journey together, I want you to keep three principles in mind:

1. **Progress, not perfection:** You don't need to transform everything overnight. Small, consistent changes compound over time into remarkable results. Start where you are, with what you have, and build from there.

2. **Listen to your body:** Your body is constantly communicating with you. Learn to hear its whispers before they become shouts. Trust your intuition about what feels right for your healing journey.

3. **Hope with action:** Hope without action is just wishful thinking. Action without hope is exhausting and unsustainable. But hope combined with action creates the possibility for miracles.

So I invite you to walk with me through the pages ahead, not as a patient, but as a partner in possibility.

You don't have to be perfect. You just need to begin.

PART *Three*

AWAKENING TO POSSIBILITY

Discovering the Path

CHAPTER 7:
BEYOND THE PHYSICAL

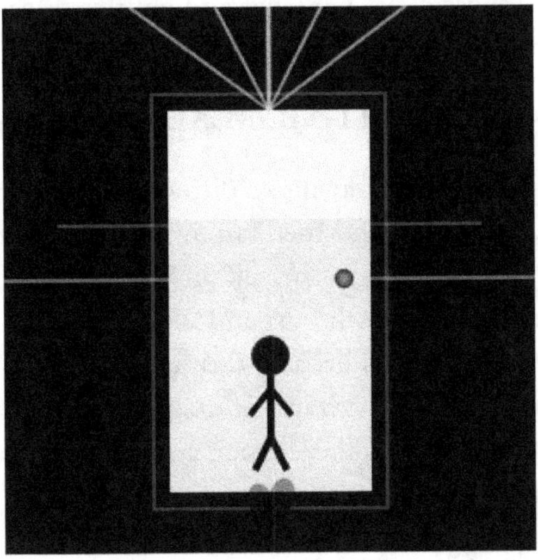

The relentless assault of surgery, chemotherapy, and radiation had left me not just physically diminished, but emotionally and spiritually hollowed out. Each day felt like a battle fought on terrain of fatigue and uncertainty. Despite rigidly following every piece of conventional medical advice, a nagging question began to surface: Was this truly all there was? Could I do more to reclaim my life, not just my health?

My entrepreneurial drive, which had helped me initially process the diagnosis with such clarity, now shifted its focus from problem-solving in business to seeking deeper answers for my healing.

SEEDS OF INQUIRY: A NEW WORLD OPENS UP

Six weeks into the conventional "standard of care," a profound realization dawned: while invaluable, this model felt incomplete. My body was being treated, but my spirit felt neglected. The treatments were attacking the cancer, but they were also attacking me. I was surviving, but was I truly healing?

During this period of intense introspection, I began actively seeking other perspectives. I devoured books and listened to specialists and researchers, but found no single, clear answer within conventional medicine. The message was consistent: we can fight this disease, extend your life, manage symptoms, but we cannot cure it.

THE SPIRITUAL REALIZATION

In parallel, I found myself drawn to a different world entirely - holistic healers, spiritual teachers, and meditation masters. I attended several meditation retreats to immerse myself in the experience, and delved into mystical traditions of both East and West. The non-duality model, often associated with what's broadly termed 'New Age' spirituality in the west, resonated deeply with me. It draws extensively from ancient wisdom traditions like Advaita Vedanta, a Hindu philosophy that had always intrigued me.

My wife's study of "A Course in Miracles" (ACIM), a text that presents similar core concepts through Christian metaphors, further opened my mind to these possibilities. Her daily practice and the peace I witnessed in her approach to my illness became a living example of these teachings in action.

I discovered modern teachers such as Eckhart Tolle, Wayne Dyer, Rupert Spira, Deepak Chopra, Bruce Lipton, and Dr. Joe Dispenza. These contemporary thinkers don't adhere to any specific religious dogma or rituals. Instead, they have meticulously studied the world's major religions and extracted the core essence of each tradition to formulate frameworks that are both understandable and practical for modern life.

THE UNIVERSAL MESSAGE

What struck me most profoundly was that Western teachers and scholars have made a tremendous contribution by seamlessly combining the best of Hinduism, Buddhism, Christianity, and mystical Sufism. We are discovering that the fundamental message across all religions is essentially the same, once you strip away the superficial layers of symbols and rituals that were necessary in their respective eras for the masses to grasp abstract spiritual concepts while surviving in harsher environments.

This convergence wasn't just intellectually satisfying; it was deeply comforting. It suggested that truth transcends cultural boundaries and that the wisdom humanity has accumulated over millennia points to common insights about consciousness, healing, and our deeper nature.

THE PARADIGM SHIFT: FROM BODY TO CONSCIOUSNESS

Slowly, painstakingly, a revolutionary idea began to take root within me: I am more than just this physical body and its transient mind. While the body's eventual decay is an undeniable truth we often avoid confronting, the essence of who I am, my consciousness, my awareness, my 'Soul', is something eternal, unbounded, and intrinsically connected to an infinite, unified field of existence.

This understanding, rooted in ancient wisdom and increasingly supported by modern science, didn't just appeal to my intuition; it resonated deeply with my logical, engineering mind. I'm never convinced unless there's sound logic behind a hypothesis. For the first time, I found a framework that explained the unseen, a hypothesis with profound implications: if my true nature was infinite consciousness, then the power to heal, to influence my physical reality, lay within me, waiting to be accessed.

THE SCIENCE BEHIND THE SPIRITUALITY

What made this shift possible for my analytical mind was discovering how quantum physics, neuroscience, and consciousness research were beginning to validate what mystics had taught for millennia. The observer effect in quantum mechanics suggests that consciousness plays a fundamental role in physical reality. When scientists observe subatomic particles, the very act of observation changes the behavior of those particles.

Neuroplasticity research shows that our thoughts literally reshape our brains. Every time we think a thought, we strengthen certain neural pathways while allowing others to weaken. This means that by changing our thinking patterns, we can literally rewire our brains for healing, optimism, and well-being.

Epigenetics reveals that our mental and emotional states can influence gene expression. Our genes are not our destiny; they are more like a hardware platform that can run different software programs depending on environmental inputs, including our thoughts, emotions, and beliefs.

This wasn't just wishful thinking; it was emerging science that suggested consciousness might be far more powerful than conventional medicine acknowledges.

CHAPTER 8:
THE DISCOVERY OF MEDITATION

You should sit in meditation for twenty minutes every day — unless you're too busy; then you should sit for an hour.
— Zen Proverb

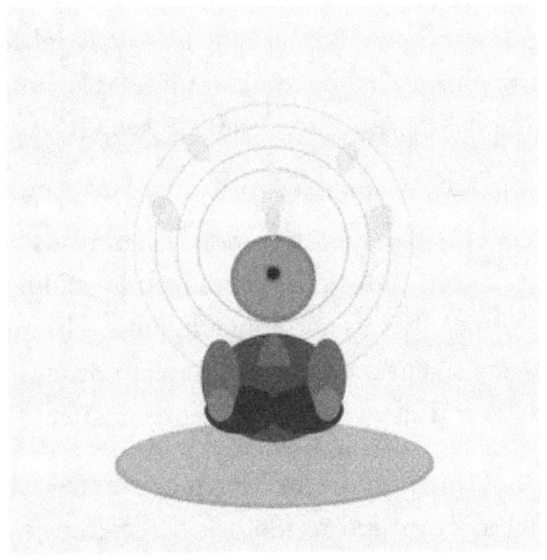

A PATH TO INNER POWER

This philosophical shift naturally led me to explore meditation as a practical means to access this inner power. I went to many retreats to learn meditation, experimented with numerous traditions: Vipassana (Buddhist), Mantra meditation (like TM and Chopra's methods), Zen, and various Indian styles. Yet, like many beginners, I struggled with the 'monkey mind', that incessant stream of distracting thoughts, past grievances, and future anxieties. My body complained too, making it difficult to sit still even for ten minutes.

The physical discomfort was particularly challenging given my weakened state from treatment. My back would ache, my legs would fall asleep, and my mind would race with worries about scan results, treatment schedules, family and business concerns. I began to wonder if meditation was just another thing I was failing at during an already difficult time.

FINDING DR. JOE DISPENZA

It was then that I encountered Dr. Joe Dispenza and his groundbreaking work, particularly his book Becoming Supernatural. Dr. Joe presented a science-based healing model that immediately appealed to my logical brain. Unlike other spiritual teachers who relied primarily on faith or ancient wisdom, Dr. Joe backed up his teachings with neuroscience, quantum physics, and measurable research.

His meditations weren't just about 'clearing your mind'; they were purposefully designed, often incorporating specific music and sound frequencies that harmonize with brain waves, gently guiding the mind into states conducive to deep focus and inner stillness. His guided voice and changing soundscapes kept me engaged, moving my awareness through my body in a way that truly quieted the mental chatter.

For me, Dr. Joe's method felt like having 'training wheels' for a beginner, yet it offered profound results for those ready to dive deep. Its direct focus on healing, whether physical or psychological, made it an indispensable tool. Here was someone who could explain exactly what was happening in my brain during meditation, why it worked, and how it could facilitate healing.

THE CANCÚN RETREAT EXPERIENCE

After viewing several of Dr. Joe's videos on YouTube, I chose to attend one of his live events. I found a week-long meditation retreat in Cancún, Mexico, and registered to further explore meditation-based healing practices. This experience would prove to be a pivotal turning point in my healing journey.

The retreat brought together about 600 people from around the world, all seeking transformation and healing. Some were dealing with cancer like me, others with chronic pain, depression, autoimmune conditions, or simply the desire to live more consciously. The diversity of the group was remarkable, doctors and teachers, entrepreneurs and artists, people from their twenties to their eighties. For the first time since my diagnosis, I felt profoundly understood without having to say a word. We were all there because we believed that a different future was possible.

Each day began at 6 AM with a meditation session, followed by breakfast and then a lecture from Dr. Joe explaining the science behind the practices. The afternoons included another meditation and often group sharing sessions where participants described their experiences and breakthroughs.

LEARNING THE SCIENCE OF TRANSFORMATION

At the retreat, I learned about the scientific aspects of Dr. Joe's meditation model in much greater detail. He explained how different brainwave states correspond to different states of consciousness and healing potential. Beta waves (14-30 Hz) are associated with normal waking consciousness and analytical thinking. Alpha waves (8-13 Hz) correspond to relaxed awareness. Theta waves (4-7 Hz) are associated with deep meditation, creativity, and healing. Delta waves (0.5-3 Hz) occur during deep sleep and unconscious states.

The goal of the meditations was to move from beta (stressed, analytical) into alpha and theta states, where the brain becomes highly plastic and open to change. In these states, we could literally rewire our neural networks, release trauma stored in the body, and access what Dr. Joe calls the "quantum field", the realm of infinite possibility that exists beyond our normal sensory experience.

UNDERSTANDING THE MIND-BODY CONNECTION

Dr. Joe taught us to understand how our bodies are guided by the interplay between the brain and mind. Think of the brain as the physical computer and the mind as its operating system, orchestrating all functions. Your thoughts are like the apps you run, each shaping your experience much like programs shape what you see on your screen.

Just as different apps yield different results, your thoughts influence your well-being. If you wish to see a healthier body, it begins with choosing and cultivating healthier thoughts, the very "app" you allow your mind to run. By learning to adjust these mental programs, you gain the ability to influence your body's responses through intentional thinking.

This wasn't just theory; it was backed by research. Studies of Dr. Joe's retreat participants showed measurable changes in gene expression, immune function, and neurotransmitter production after just one week of intensive meditation practice.

FIRST MEDITATION BREAKTHROUGH: A PROFOUND AWAKENING

In the days following the Cancún retreat, as I continued Dr. Joe's meditation practices at home, my conviction deepened: this was the right healing path for me.

The essence of meditation is withdrawing from sensory input—light, sound, touch, taste, smell—so your attention becomes fully absorbed in a single point of focus. Dr. Joe's method is designed precisely for this. You wear an eye mask to block light and noise-canceling headphones to listen to guided meditations set to specially composed music. With external distractions eliminated, your brain tunes into the binaural frequencies embedded in the soundtrack while following Dr. Joe's guided instructions.

I established a dedicated meditation space in our home, a quiet corner with a comfortable chair, where I could sit undisturbed each morning or at night. I began with 30-minute sessions and gradually worked up to 60-90 minutes as my ability to maintain focus improved.

THE VOID EXPERIENCE

During one particular session about three weeks after returning from Mexico, we were guided to direct our awareness to the infinite darkness of the void, a space where nothing exists. It took several minutes to settle in, relax my body completely, and visualize this emptiness.

The aim was to let go of all thoughts and become aware of pure being, just yourself, and nothing else. When you reach this state, only pure consciousness remains, stripped of all external layers. In this non-physical realm, you can merge with the void.

THE DISSOLUTION

At that moment, something extraordinary happened. I felt myself, the familiar body-mind identity that I had always assumed was "me", completely dissolve, like a drop of water merging into an endless ocean. There was no longer a sense of being located in a physical body or even having a separate identity.

Instead, there was just pure awareness, vast, peaceful, and completely without boundaries. I wasn't experiencing this state; I was this state. The distinction between observer and observed had completely disappeared.

BEYOND WORDS

The experience was profound beyond words. I had never known such peace and joy; tears of happiness streamed down my face when I eventually returned to normal consciousness. Some might call it love, or a sense of unity with the universe. Others might describe it as touching the face of God. Whatever you call it, it was truly transformative.

The peace wasn't just an absence of anxiety or stress; it was a positive presence, a deep knowing that all was well, that I was held and loved by something infinitely greater than my small personal self. For perhaps the first time in my life, I understood what spiritual teachers meant when they talked about unconditional love.

THE SHIFT IN PERSPECTIVE

From that point on, I knew I needed to embrace this practice whole-heartedly. The experience had shown me that healing wasn't something I needed to struggle and fight for. Instead, it would unfold naturally and effortlessly when I aligned myself with this deeper truth of who I am.

My only task was to return to this state regularly through meditation, to enjoy the journey, and to trust the process completely.

CHAPTER 9:
CHOOSING THE NATURAL PATH

Nature does not hurry, yet everything is accomplished.
— Lao Tzu

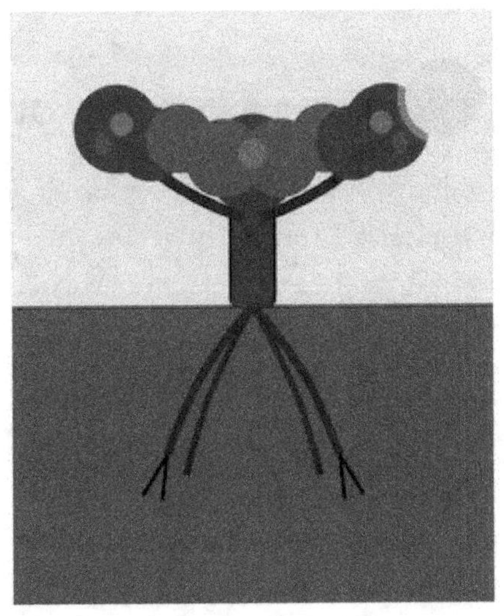

INVESTIGATING ALTERNATIVES: A DELIBERATE CHOICE

Right after my diagnosis, my wife and I immediately plunged into researching everything we could find on brain cancer, specifically Glioblastoma. At that time, there wasn't a vast amount of readily available published material online compared to today. Still, we learned a tremendous amount about neuroscience, how the brain functions, the intricate behavior of cancer cells, and their reliance on glucose for fuel.

We spent countless hours reading medical journals, watching scientific presentations, and following leads from one expert to another. We learned about the blood-brain barrier and why so few treatments can effectively reach brain tumors. We studied cancer metabolism and discovered how cancer cells consume glucose at rates 10-50 times higher than normal cells.

We consulted numerous doctors and specialists beyond our primary team. Some recommended cocktails of FDA-approved drugs originally designed for other ailments, like hypertension medication that showed some promise in small studies, or antidepressants that might have anti-cancer properties. However, these all came with serious side effects, and I quickly felt that pursuing such experimental combinations was not for me.

EXPLORING INTERNATIONAL OPTIONS

We explored many clinics outside the US offering adjuvant therapies. Germany has several clinics offering hyperthermia treatment, mistletoe therapy, and other alternative approaches. Mexico has facilities providing high-dose vitamin C infusions, ozone therapy, and experimental immunotherapies. Switzerland offers clinics combining conventional and alternative treatments.

Most of these were experimental, exorbitantly expensive (often $50,000-$100,000 for a month of treatment), and not covered by insurance. Crucially, they were generally not regulated or approved by reputable hospitals or universities. The success stories were anecdotal, and the scientific evidence was often limited or non-existent.

We discovered that there was essentially no safe, proven cure for brain cancer available beyond the "standard of care" model followed by most doctors and hospitals in the US. While many clinical trials for new Glioblastoma drugs were underway, none had yet proven broadly effective.

CLINICAL TRIAL REJECTION

I even tried to enroll in several clinical trials myself, but was rejected because I had two cancers simultaneously. Clinical trials require very specific patient populations to generate meaningful data, and my unique situation would have made it impossible to determine which outcomes were related to the brain cancer versus the bladder cancer.

This rejection was initially disappointing but ultimately liberating. It forced me to take complete responsibility for my healing rather than hoping that some external treatment would save me.

THE OPTUNE DEVICE DECISION

For GBM treatment, there is an electrical device called Optune that delivers low-intensity alternating electrical fields to the brain where the tumor is located. These Tumor Treating Fields (TTFields) are designed to disrupt rapidly dividing cancer cells.

The device must be worn continuously, at least 18 hours per day, with adhesive patches applied to a shaved scalp, connected to a portable battery pack that weighs several pounds. The scalp needs to be shaved every few days to ensure good contact with the arrays, which are replaced regularly. The most common side effect is skin irritation, but some patients also experience fatigue and other complications.

My radiation oncologist recommended Optune with enthusiasm, calling it a breakthrough in GBM treatment. When I asked about the projected life extension from such a demanding regimen, his answer was candidly "perhaps another six months, maybe a year if we're lucky."

For me, that was a non-starter. The idea of living out my final months tethered to a machine, looking like a medical experiment, dealing with constant skin irritation and the weight of carrying batteries everywhere, felt like an unacceptable compromise on quality of life. I could see myself becoming defined by the device, unable to swim, shower normally, or even hug my family without being conscious of the equipment.

I chose to live fully, however long that might be, rather than endure prolonged medical dependency.

MAKING THE NATURAL CHOICE

In the end, with this newfound clarity, we made a definitive choice: to focus entirely on natural, self-directed methods for healing. If that meant accepting a shorter lifespan, I was perfectly okay with it. My focus shifted from merely extending life to optimizing life, making whatever time I had as meaningful, joyful, and authentic as possible.

This wasn't a rejection of all conventional medicine, surgery had saved my life by removing the bulk of the tumor. But it was a conscious choice to pursue healing rather than just disease management, to focus on building health rather than just fighting illness.

EMBRACING SPIRITUALITY: A REDEFINED EXISTENCE

Cancer forces an undeniable confrontation with mortality. While most of us live busy lives skirting this ultimate truth, my diagnosis presented a 'Come to Jesus' moment, stripping away all pretense and forcing me to look death squarely in the eye. My family upbringing, with its spiritual roots, undoubtedly helped me come to terms with the ephemeral nature of human existence.

But this wasn't just an intellectual exercise. The fear of death, when you're actually facing it, is primal and overwhelming. I had to work through waves of terror about leaving my wife alone, about missing my children's future milestones, about all the experiences I would never have. These fears would hit me at unexpected moments, while brushing my teeth, during a business meeting, while watching a sunset. My wife, ever my partner in this journey, took my hand and said, 'Then this is the path we will walk.' In that moment, I knew I wasn't choosing this alone.

THE PHILOSOPHICAL QUEST

With mortality knocking, my long-standing, albeit peripheral, interest in philosophy and religion transformed into an urgent quest. As a hard-charging entrepreneur, I'd previously lacked time for such 'esoteric' pursuits. Now, the questions that had always lingered in the background demanded answers: What is the purpose of human existence? What happens after we die? What is the true nature of reality? How do we explain consciousness, the soul, the unseen forces that seem to underpin everything?

My YouTube feed became a virtual university, featuring lectures from acclaimed scientists like Dr. Bruce Lipton and Dr. Rupert Sheldrake, philosophers like Sam Harris and Alan Watts, and spiritual teachers like Eckhart Tolle, Wayne Dyer, and Krishnamurti. I read voraciously, everything from ancient Buddhist texts to cutting-edge consciousness research.

THE CONVERGENCE OF WISDOM

What struck me most was the astonishing convergence of wisdom traditions: the core messages of Buddhism, Hinduism, and Christian mysticism, stripped of their cultural trappings, revealed strikingly similar truths. They all pointed to the same fundamental insights: consciousness is primary, separation is an illusion, love is the fundamental force of the universe, and death is a transformation rather than an ending.

The symbols and language that once made scriptures impenetrable now seemed like necessary tools for their original audiences, meant to convey abstract spiritual concepts in relatable forms. Jesus talking about the "Kingdom of Heaven within," Buddha teaching about the "Buddha nature," and Hindu sages describing "Atman" (the individual soul) as identical to "Brahman" (universal consciousness)—they were all pointing to the same truth.

SCIENCE MEETS SPIRITUALITY

In parallel, I immersed myself in quantum physics, biology, and neuroscience, seeking to understand physical reality through a scientific lens. I began to witness how science, in its relentless inquiry, was echoing ancient mystical teachings.

Quantum entanglement suggests that particles can be instantaneously connected across vast distances, supporting the mystical insight of fundamental unity. The measurement problem in quantum mechanics implies that consciousness plays a role in creating physical reality. Studies of near-death experiences reveal remarkably consistent reports of expanded consciousness during clinical death.

This integration of science and spirituality became a cohesive, understandable framework. And in this process, I discovered enormous joy and profound peace in peeling back the layers to understand who I truly am, a truth that wisdom traditions have whispered for millennia.

OVERCOMING CHALLENGES: RESILIENCE AND THE POWER OF ACCEPTANCE

The path of self-directed healing is not a straight line; it's a winding journey with inevitable detours, setbacks, and unexpected challenges. There were days when old habits threatened to resurface, moments when fear and uncertainty, particularly the fear of recurrence, resurfaced like an unwelcome shadow.

Some mornings I would wake up feeling perfectly fine, only to be hit by a wave of anxiety about whether the cancer was growing back. Other days, a headache or moment of forgetfulness would send me into a spiral of worry, wondering if these were signs that the treatment had failed.

THE SUPPORT SYSTEM

In these moments, my wife and family's unwavering support was not just crucial; it was my lifeline. Their belief in me, even when my own resolve wavered, enabled me to accept these setbacks as part of the process rather than failures, and to keep moving forward.

My wife became particularly skilled at recognizing when I was spiraling into anxiety and would gently remind me to return to my true being, in the present moment, to the practices that had brought me peace. She never dismissed my fears, but she also never let me stay stuck in them.

THE POWER OF RADICAL ACCEPTANCE

The most profound shift came with radical acceptance and surrender. By consciously releasing all resistance to what is, even the terrifying prospect of death, a profound sense of freedom began to emerge.

When I genuinely became okay with whatever outcome unfolded, the crippling grip of fear, worry, and anxiety began to dissolve. This wasn't resignation or giving up; it was a deep trust in the intelligence of the universe and my place within it.

This liberation redirected immense energy and attention, no longer consumed by internal struggle, but now available for the work of true healing.

A TRANSFORMED RELATIONSHIP WITH MORTALITY

This journey significantly lessened my fear of death, a profoundly difficult yet ultimately liberating step, especially for someone with deep family responsibilities. Through exploring timeless wisdom that posits life beyond the physical body and mind, my perception of mortality transformed.

I began to see death not as an ending, but as a transition, like taking off a heavy coat that you no longer need. The essential "me", consciousness itself, couldn't be destroyed any more than space could be destroyed. This wasn't just a comforting belief; it felt like a direct knowing that emerged from my meditation experiences.

While I acknowledge this perspective may not resonate with everyone's beliefs, for me, it was transformational, allowing me to live more fully in the present moment rather than being paralyzed by future fears.

Even Einstein, one of the greatest scientific minds in history, described death as simply "a change of address in space-time." That idea resonated deeply with me. The fear of death hasn't vanished entirely, but it has slowly receded into the background—no longer the constant shadow it once was, but a quiet presence I've learned to live alongside.

THE GIFT OF PRESENCE

With the fear of death diminished, I found myself able to be truly present in ways I never had before. Colors seemed more vivid, conversations more meaningful, simple pleasures more profound. Food tasted better. Sunsets were more beautiful. Hugs with my family felt like sacred experiences. Before, a hug might have been a brief, almost automatic gesture on the way out the door. Now, it was a moment of profound connection, a silent acknowledgment of how precious our time together truly was.

This wasn't about denial or forced positivity; it was about removing the veil of anxiety that had colored my perception for so long. When you're not constantly worried about the future or regretful about the past, the present moment reveals its extraordinary richness.

MY HOLISTIC HEALING PLAN: A NEW WAY OF LIVING

Armed with this new understanding, my wife and I collaborated to design a comprehensive plan for self-healing, a radical departure from the conventional approach. This wasn't merely a set of adjustments; it was a conscious, daily commitment to a new way of living built on eight foundational pillars:

Mindfulness & Meditation -- Embarking on a consistent daily meditation practice to calm the nervous system, release deeply held stress, and cultivate inner peace. This became my primary medicine, practiced for 1-2 hours each morning.

Nourishing Diet -- Transitioning to a plant-based ketogenic approach, meticulously eliminating sugar and minimizing carbohydrates to starve cancer cells while supporting cellular health.

Physical Movement -- Integrating daily exercise and activity, listening to my body's needs while promoting circulation, energy, and overall vitality.

Restorative Sleep -- Prioritizing eight hours of quality sleep each night, recognizing its critical role in cellular repair and immune function.

Targeted Nutrition -- Incorporating a carefully selected regimen of supplements to ensure optimal nutrient intake, supporting my body's healing mechanisms.

Positive Mindset Cultivation -- Actively leveraging the power of positive thinking, visualization, and optimistic self-talk to influence my internal landscape.

Environmental Purge -- Setting firm boundaries to consciously reduce stress in my home and work life, actively avoiding negative influences.

Radical Acceptance & Surrender -- Practicing radical acceptance of whatever transpired, releasing resistance, fear, worry, and the need to control outcomes. Cultivating deep surrender to a Higher Intelligence, trusting in what was meant for my highest good.

This comprehensive transformation taught me that healing isn't just about eliminating disease; it's about creating a life so vibrant and meaningful that illness simply cannot take root.

PART *Four*

THE MEDS FOUNDATION

Building the Four Pillars

CHAPTER 10:
UNDERSTANDING MEDS

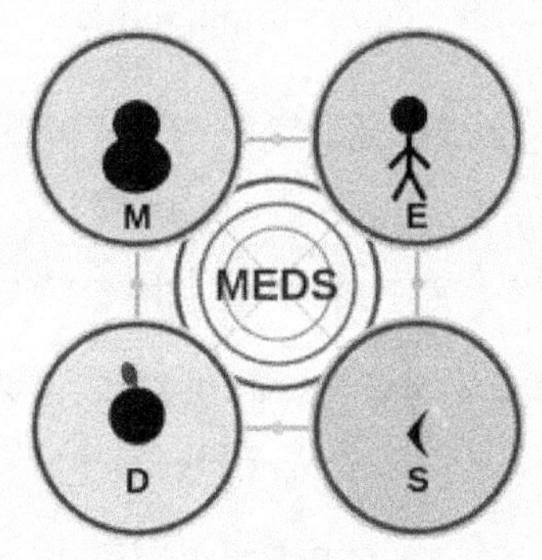

After months of research, experimentation, and deep introspection following my diagnosis, I began to see a pattern emerging in what truly moved the needle in my healing. While conventional medicine had given me time by removing the tumor, it was becoming clear that real healing—the kind that transforms you from the inside out—required something more comprehensive.

What emerged from my journey was not a random collection of wellness practices, but four foundational pillars that, when practiced together, created a synergistic effect far greater than any single intervention. I came to call this framework MEDS: Meditation, Exercise, Diet, and Sleep. I later discovered that other wellness practitioners have independently arrived at similar frameworks using the same acronym—

which only reinforced my belief that these four pillars represent something fundamental about how human beings heal.

The acronym MEDS was intentional. Just as conventional medicine offers meds (medications) to treat symptoms, I was creating my own 'meds'—a prescription for healing that addressed not just the physical manifestation of disease, but its roots in mind, body, and spirit.

WHY THESE FOUR PILLARS?

Through my research and personal experience, I discovered that each of these pillars addresses a critical aspect of healing:

1. **Meditation** rewires the brain, reduces stress hormones, and connects us to our deeper healing intelligence

2. **Exercise** moves lymph, oxygenates tissues, and signals to the body that we choose life

3. **Diet** provides the raw materials for cellular repair while starving disease

4. **Sleep** provides the critical restoration time when the body heals, the immune system strengthens, and cellular repair occurs

What I discovered was that these weren't just helpful additions to conventional treatment—they were fundamental to creating an internal environment where healing could occur. Each pillar supported and amplified the others in remarkable ways.

THE SYNERGY OF MEDS

When I meditated, I found it easier to make healthy food choices. When I ate well, I had more energy for gentle exercise. When I moved my body, I felt more connected spiritually. When I nurtured my spiritual connection, meditation became deeper and more profound. It was a virtuous cycle, each practice reinforcing and strengthening the others.

This interconnection wasn't just my subjective experience. Science was beginning to understand these connections too. Meditation has been shown to influence gene expression and immune function. Exercise triggers the release of brain-derived neurotrophic factor (BDNF), which supports neural health. Diet directly impacts the gut microbiome, which produces neurotransmitters that affect mood and cognition. Spiritual practices have been linked to longer telomeres and improved stress resilience.

FROM CRISIS MANAGEMENT TO LIFESTYLE

Initially, MEDS was my crisis response—a desperate attempt to throw everything I could at cancer. But as weeks turned to months, something shifted. These practices stopped feeling like treatments and started feeling like a way of life. They weren't things I had to do; they became things I wanted to do, things that made me feel more alive, more present, more myself.

The beauty of MEDS is its accessibility. You don't need expensive equipment or exotic supplements. You don't need to travel to distant clinics or undergo complex procedures. Everything you need is already within you—MEDS simply provides the framework to activate your body's innate healing wisdom.

A LIVING FRAMEWORK

MEDS isn't rigid or prescriptive. It's a living framework that adapts to where you are in your journey. Some days, meditation might be just five minutes of conscious breathing. Exercise might be a gentle walk to the mailbox. Diet might be simply choosing water over soda. Spirituality might be a moment of gratitude before sleep.

The key is consistency, not perfection. It's about gently, persistently nurturing all four pillars, understanding that they work together to create something greater than the sum of their parts.

In the chapters that follow, we'll explore each pillar in detail—not as abstract concepts, but as practical, applicable practices that you can begin implementing today. Whether you're facing a health crisis or simply seeking to optimize your wellbeing, MEDS offers a roadmap to transformation that honors both ancient wisdom and modern science.

CHAPTER 11:
MEDITATION — THE MIND'S MEDICINE

Meditation is not a means to an end.
It is both the means and the end.
—Jiddu Krishnamurti

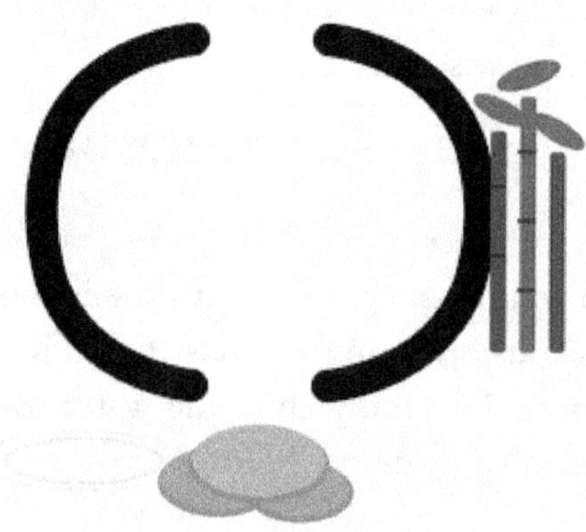

Of all the pillars in MEDS, meditation was perhaps the most transformative—and initially, the most challenging. As an entrepreneur accustomed to solving problems through action, sitting still and 'doing nothing' felt counterintuitive, even wasteful. But what I discovered was that meditation isn't doing nothing; it's doing the most important something—rewiring the very operating system of healing.

THE SCIENCE THAT CONVINCED ME

My analytical mind needed evidence, and I found it in abundance. Studies showed that regular meditation could:

1. Reduce inflammatory markers like C-reactive protein and interleukin-6

2. Increase telomerase activity, potentially slowing cellular aging

3. Boost natural killer cell activity, enhancing immune surveillance

4. Alter gene expression in ways that support healing

5. Reduce cortisol and other stress hormones that suppress immune function

This wasn't just relaxation—it was a powerful medical intervention that required no prescription, had no side effects, and cost nothing.

MY DAILY PRACTICE

I developed a meditation practice that evolved with my capacity. In the beginning, during the worst of treatment, five minutes felt like an eternity. My body ached, my mind raced with fears, and sitting still felt like torture. But I persisted, gently, without judgment.

My morning routine became sacred:

6:00 AM: Wake up naturally, no alarm

6:30 AM: Begin meditation, starting with breath awareness

6:30-7:30 AM: Deeper meditation using Dr. Joe Dispenza's techniques

7:30 AM: Gratitude practice and intention setting for the day

Some days I slept in, because rest had become a priority. On those mornings, my routine shifted accordingly. When sleep eluded me entirely—or when I found myself wide awake at 3 a.m.—I would first try a silent meditation lying down. If that didn't ease me back to sleep, I'd get out of bed, put on my headphones, and dive into a full hour-long meditation session. Afterward, if I felt sleepy, I'd simply go back to sleep.

I recognize this flexibility isn't available to everyone. If you have an early work schedule or young children who need your attention, you'll need to adapt these practices to fit your reality. The principles matter more than the precise routine.

THE TECHNIQUES THAT WORKED

Through experimentation, I found several meditation approaches particularly powerful for healing:

Body Scanning: Moving awareness through each part of my body, sending love and healing energy to every cell. This helped me reconnect with my body as an ally rather than an enemy.

Visualization: Imagining white light flooding the areas where tumors had been, seeing healthy cells thriving, picturing my immune system as powerful and intelligent.

The Void: Learning to rest in pure awareness, beyond thought, beyond fear, beyond the identity of 'cancer patient.' In this space, I wasn't sick—I simply was.

Loving-Kindness: Sending compassion to myself, to my family, to other patients, even to the cancer cells themselves. This practice dissolved the internal war and created space for healing.

OVERCOMING THE OBSTACLES

The path wasn't smooth. Some days, meditation felt impossible. Pain, nausea, or anxiety would dominate. On these days, I learned to be gentle with myself. Even one conscious breath was meditation. Even a moment of presence was victory.

I discovered that the 'perfect' meditation doesn't exist. Some sessions were profound, filled with insights and deep peace. Others were struggles, wrestling with monkey mind for every second. Both were equally valuable. The struggle sessions taught me patience and persistence. The peaceful ones showed me what was possible.

THE RIPPLE EFFECTS

As my meditation practice deepened, its effects rippled through every aspect of my life. I became less reactive to stressful news or difficult emotions. I could observe pain without being consumed by it. Fear still arose, but it no longer controlled me.

Most remarkably, meditation changed my relationship with the illness itself. Cancer stopped being an enemy to defeat and became a teacher showing me how to live more consciously. This shift from resistance to acceptance, from fighting to flowing, created an internal environment where healing could naturally unfold.

CHAPTER 12:
EXERCISE — MOVEMENT AS LIFE

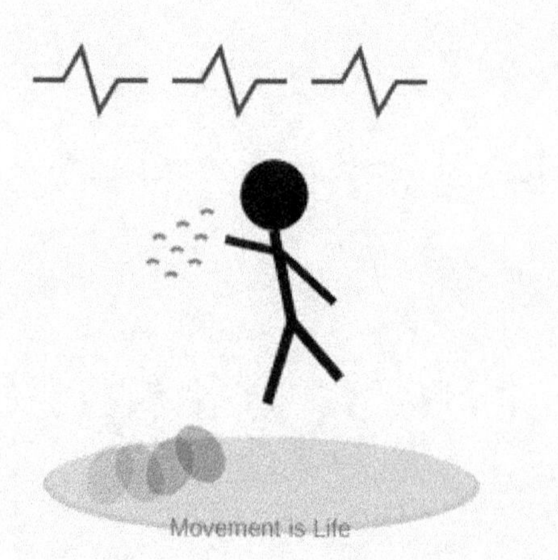

There is a moment in every healing journey when the body begins whispering: I want to move again.

At first, it's subtle, an easing of stiffness, a slight increase in energy, a spark of restlessness after weeks or months of stillness. Then the whisper becomes a gentle pull, a nudge toward reclaiming the physical self that illness, fatigue, and treatment had temporarily taken away.

Movement, I learned, is not just exercise. It is communication. It is a dialogue with your body, a process of relearning what strength feels like, what fatigue means, and how resilience rebuilds itself slowly, quietly, one breath and one step at a time.

WHY MOVEMENT IS CRUCIAL FOR THE IMMUNE SYSTEM

When I was at my weakest, movement seemed counterintuitive. I believed rest equaled recovery. And while rest is essential, I discovered that stillness in excess can slow healing, weaken immunity, and dull the body's natural rhythms.

The lymphatic system does not have a pump like the heart. It relies on muscle contraction to circulate lymph fluid, which carries immune cells, detoxifies waste, and helps fight infection. When the body is sedentary for long periods, lymph flow becomes stagnant.

Gentle movement—walking, stretching, light yoga—activates this system, helping the body's inner defenses stay awake, alert, and responsive.

EXERCISE DURING AND AFTER TREATMENT

At the beginning of my recovery, the idea of 'exercise' felt almost unpleasant. How could I exercise when my body was swollen, exhausted, and fighting battles deep inside me?

The truth is, exercise during and after treatment does not look like the fitness you see in gyms or on social media. It looks like presence. It looks like curiosity. It looks like honoring your limits without abandoning your potential.

I began with micro-movements:

1. Slow walks around the room

2. Stretching my arms overhead

3. Gentle neck rotations

4. Breathing while lifting my chest

Walking became my anchor. Some days I could walk only five minutes. Other days, twenty. I let my body decide.

THE 10% RULE

I never increased activity drastically. Instead, I added about 10% at a time—10% longer, 10% more repetitions, 10% more intensity. This gradual progression protected my joints, my stamina, and my emotional health.

During this phase, I became a student of my own body. Signs that I needed to slow down included dizziness, nausea, shortness of breath, chest pressure, neuropathy flares, excessive fatigue hours after activity, and brain fog worsening immediately after exercise.

MANAGING CHEMO BRAIN AND NEUROPATHY

Two of the most frustrating side effects of treatment were chemo brain—the cognitive fog, slow recall, and difficulty focusing—and neuropathy—the tingling and numbness in my feet.

For chemo brain, I found that movement stimulated bilateral brain integration. Walking, which naturally alternates left and right movements, helped clear mental fog. Balancing exercises activated the cerebellum and improved focus.

For neuropathy, gentle movements helped: foot rotations, hand-flexing and wrist circles, massaging hands and feet, rolling my feet on a small ball, and walking barefoot on soft surfaces to stimulate nerve endings.

Movement restored circulation. Circulation restored sensation. Sensation restored confidence.

REBUILDING STRENGTH

As I gained energy, I slowly introduced strength training—bodyweight squats, wall push-ups, and light resistance bands. Muscle loss is common during cancer treatment, and rebuilding it restored not only physical strength but emotional confidence.

The first time I could walk around the block, I felt really happy. Not because it was dramatic, but because I felt my body returning to me. Movement became a declaration: I am still here. I am still capable. I am still choosing life.

CHAPTER 13:
DIET — FOOD AS MEDICINE

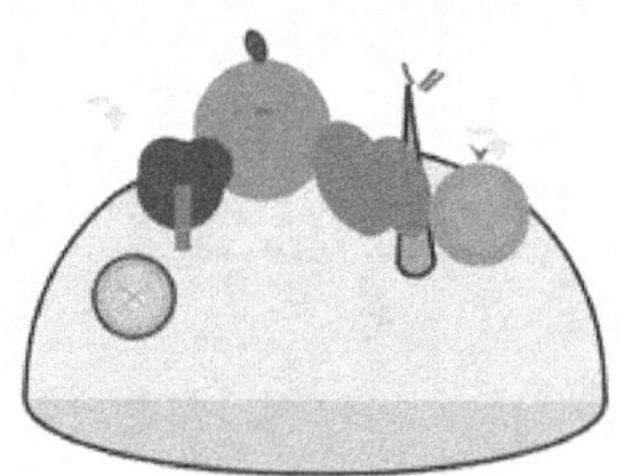

Healing is never one-dimensional. It is not confined to scans, surgeries, or treatments. It is a full-body symphony, one where every organ, every cell, every thought participates. And one of the most powerful conductors in that symphony is the food we choose to place on our plate.

During my own journey, I discovered that nutrition is not simply about calories or macronutrients. It is about energy and vibration. It is about inflammation and repair. It is about supporting the body the way a parent supports a recovering child: with gentleness, consistency, and patience.

THE ANTI-INFLAMMATORY KITCHEN

Inflammation is a word we often hear but rarely understand. In the simplest terms, chronic inflammation is the body stuck in 'alarm mode,' even when there is no emergency. For someone navigating cancer, treatment, recovery, or chronic illness, inflammation becomes one of the invisible enemies.

When I learned this, I realized that my kitchen needed to transform from a convenience space into a healing sanctuary. I began to see each food as either an accelerator of inflammation or an ally against it.

The first shift was removing as many processed products as possible. Packaged snacks, refined sugars, seed oils, and artificial sweeteners were all whispering forms of inflammation. Instead, I shifted toward whole foods—foods that came from the earth, not factories.

THE CANCER-GLUCOSE CONNECTION

One of the most powerful motivations for dietary change came from understanding cancer biology. Cancer cells consume glucose at rates 10-50 times higher than normal cells. This isn't just a preference—it's an addiction. PET scans actually work by tracking radioactive glucose to find tumors because cancer cells grab it so aggressively.

Learning this, I couldn't justify feeding my enemy. Sugar had to go. Not completely—rigidity has its own toxicity—but dramatically. My beloved desserts, my morning sweetened coffee, my afternoon snacks—all transformed or eliminated.

Sugar = Poison. Eliminate It.

It's simple… sugar = inflammation = cardiovascular disease = cancer fuel = accelerated aging.

It hijacks your dopamine system like cocaine. A 10-day sugar fast can reset your palate and cravings. Monitor your glucose with a CGM (continuous glucose monitor) and you'll discover which foods spike your sugar level. When you change what you eat, you change which genes get expressed. That should be powerful for you.

MY ANTI-CANCER PLATE

My diet became predominantly plant-based, not from ideology but from how my body responded. A typical day looked like:

Morning: Warm lemon water, followed by green tea rich in EGCG (a powerful antioxidant)

Breakfast: A smoothie with spinach, blueberries, pumpkin seeds, hemp seeds, or chia seeds, almonds, walnuts for protein, and fruit like banana added to it. Sometimes, I would keep it real simple—blueberries, raspberries, full fat yogurt or Greek yogurt with hemp seeds

Lunch: Large salad with mixed greens, cruciferous vegetables, nuts, seeds, and olive oil dressing. Flax seeds or flax oil, MCT oil are also great add ons to your salad plate.

Dinner: Vegetable curry or soup with turmeric and ginger, served with quinoa or cauliflower rice

Snacks: Handful of raw almonds, fresh vegetables with hummus,

Figs, dates, and prunes for dessert

If I have a heavy lunch, I skip dinner and opt for Golden Milk— whole organic A2 milk boiled with turmeric, black pepper, and cardamom. I enjoy it with a few almonds or walnuts and figs or dates as a dessert substitute. If regular milk does not suit you, almond, coconut, or oat milk can be used instead.

THE POWER OF SPECIFIC FOODS

Certain foods became daily medicine:

1. **Turmeric:** With black pepper to enhance absorption, for its powerful anti-inflammatory curcumin. Golden Milk with curcumin,

black pepper and cardamom, makes a tasty bedtime drink that helps you sleep better

2. **Garlic:** Crushed and allowed to sit before cooking to activate allicin

3. **Green tea:** 3-4 cups daily for its catechins

4. **Mushrooms:** Especially shiitake and maitake for immune support

5. **Berries:** Daily, for their anthocyanins and low glycemic impact

HYDRATION AS HEALING

I had never thought of water as part of my diet, only drinking when thirsty. As a heavy coffee drinker, I rarely felt thirsty. After researching the role of hydration in cellular health and toxin elimination, I realized this oversight may have contributed to my illness.

I began drinking half my body weight in ounces each day—about 80 ounces of pure, filtered water. The improvement in my energy levels and mental clarity was noticeable within days.

INTUITIVE EATING DURING TREATMENT

Perhaps the most profound shift was learning to eat intuitively. During treatment, your body changes daily. What feels good one week can feel unbearable the next. I began listening not just to hunger, but to subtle signals.

Some days I wanted warm soups. Other days, raw vegetables. Sometimes all I wanted was fruit. I stopped labeling foods as 'good' or 'bad.' Instead, I asked: Does this support my energy? Does this calm my body? Does this align with how I want to feel? Does this help my body or help cancer cells to grow rapidly?

Food became one of my greatest teachers. It taught me patience. It taught me presence. It taught me that healing is a partnership between what you consume and how you care for yourself.

CHAPTER 14:
SLEEP — THE FOUNDATION OF HEALING

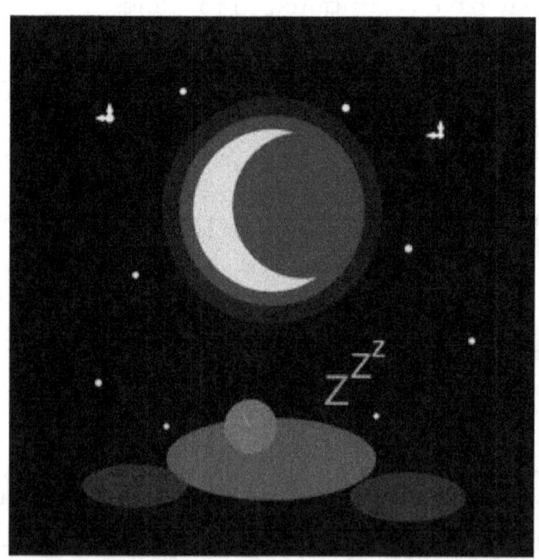

If meditation trains the mind, exercise strengthens the body, and diet provides the fuel, then sleep is the foundation upon which all healing occurs. It's the fourth pillar of MEDS, and in many ways, the most critical—because without quality sleep, the other three pillars cannot function optimally.

For most of my adult life, I treated sleep as negotiable—something to sacrifice when work demanded more hours or when there was one more thing to accomplish. Cancer taught me that sleep is not optional. It is sacred medicine.

WHY SLEEP IS NON-NEGOTIABLE FOR HEALING

During sleep, the body performs critical maintenance that cannot happen while we're awake. The brain clears out metabolic waste through the glymphatic system. The immune system produces infection-fighting cells and antibodies. Tissues repair, hormones rebalance, and memories consolidate. Without quality sleep, healing simply cannot occur optimally.

Sleep also triggers the release of melatonin, a powerful antioxidant that has been shown to inhibit tumor growth. Poor sleep, on the other hand, elevates cortisol and other stress hormones that suppress immune function and create inflammation—the very conditions that allow cancer to thrive.

THE SLEEP CRISIS DURING TREATMENT

Yet sleep was one of the first casualties of my treatment. Chemotherapy disrupted my circadian rhythm. Anxiety kept my mind racing. Night sweats and nausea made rest nearly impossible. I was trying to heal while deprived of the very process that enables healing.

This created a vicious cycle: the treatment made me too sick to sleep well, and the lack of sleep made me less able to tolerate the treatment and fight the cancer. Breaking this cycle became one of my most important battles.

CREATING A SLEEP SANCTUARY

We created what we called a "sleep sanctuary"—a cool, completely dark room with comfortable bedding, no electronic devices, and calming scents like lavender. We established a consistent bedtime routine that signaled to my body that it was time to heal.

I had to become militant about sleep hygiene:

1. **No screens after 8 PM**—the blue light suppresses melatonin production

2. **Bedroom temperature at 65-68°F**—cooler temperatures promote deeper sleep

3. **Complete darkness**—even small lights from devices disrupt circadian rhythms

4. **Consistent sleep schedule**—same bedtime and wake time every day, even weekends

5. **Magnesium supplement**—helps relax muscles and calm the nervous system

6. **Meditation before bed**—shifts brainwaves toward sleep states

7. **No caffeine after noon**—its effects last longer than most people realize

8. **Calming teas**—chamomile, valerian, or passionflower before bed. Ashwagandha supplement is also known to calm down and reduce stress, take it before going to bed

These weren't just good habits—they were non-negotiable healing practices.

THE SCIENCE OF SLEEP AND HEALING

Research has confirmed what I experienced firsthand. During deep sleep:

- The immune system produces the most white blood cells, your cancer-fighting army - Human growth hormone is released, essential for tissue repair - The brain consolidates memories and processes emotional experiences - Cellular repair and regeneration peak - Inflammation markers decrease

Studies have shown that people who consistently sleep less than six hours have significantly higher rates of cancer, heart disease, and cognitive decline. Sleep deprivation literally shortens your life—and when you're fighting cancer, you cannot afford to give the disease any advantage.

GUIDED SLEEP MEDITATIONS

One of my most valuable tools was guided sleep meditations. When anxiety made my mind race at bedtime, these recordings gave my thoughts something positive to focus on. I found meditations specifically designed for healing during sleep, with visualizations of my body repairing itself and my immune system growing stronger.

Some nights, I would listen to body scan meditations that progressively relaxed each muscle group. Other nights, I used binaural beats designed to guide brainwaves into delta sleep states. The key was having options for whatever my mind needed that particular night.

THE TRANSFORMATION

When sleep improved, everything else improved: energy, mood, mental clarity, and most importantly, immune function. I could feel my body's healing capacity expanding when I was well-rested. Treatments were easier to tolerate. My outlook was more positive. The other pillars of MEDS—meditation, exercise, and diet—all became more effective when built on a foundation of quality sleep.

Sleep became not just a health practice but a form of self-respect. Every night, as I settled into my sleep sanctuary, I was making a statement: my healing matters. My body deserves rest. Tomorrow, I will wake up stronger than today.

What began as four practical pillars was becoming something much deeper—a complete philosophy of healing that Part Five explores in full.

PART *Five*

THE EVOLUTION

From MEDS to Mind-Body-Spirit

CHAPTER 15:
THE TRANSFORMATION

We must be willing to let go of the life we planned so as to have the life that is waiting for us.
— **Joseph Campbell**

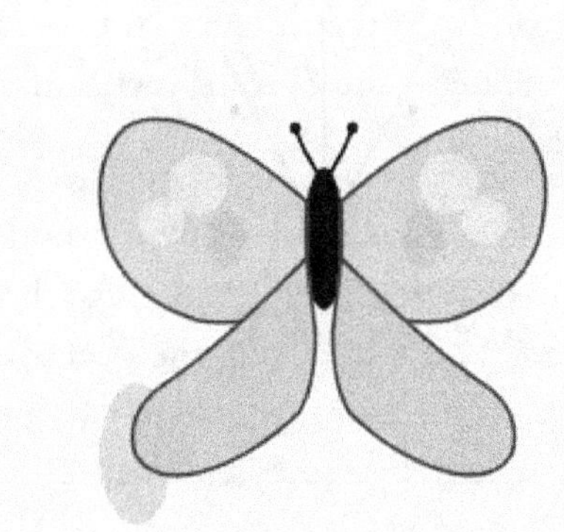

As I progressed on my healing journey, the four pillars of MEDS—Meditation, Exercise, Diet, and Sleep—began to reveal themselves as something more profound. What started as practical interventions evolved into a deeper understanding of healing that encompassed my entire being. The MEDS framework had helped me survive and live, but I felt that life is much more than just survival. It had been the perfect entry point. But now I was ready to see the bigger picture.

The transformation wasn't sudden. It was like watching the sun rise—gradual, inevitable, and transformative. As I practiced MEDS daily, I began to see that these weren't just four separate practices but expressions of three fundamental dimensions of human existence: Mind, Body, and Spirit.

THE THREE DIMENSIONS REVEALED

The shift in understanding came through direct experience. During meditation, I wasn't just calming my thoughts—I was actively reshaping my mental landscape. Exercise wasn't just moving muscles—it was honoring my body as a sacred vessel. Diet wasn't just nutrition—it was a form of self-respect and cellular communication. And spirituality wasn't just belief—it was the thread that wove everything together into meaning.

I realized that Meditation was primarily working on the Mind dimension, though it touched all three. Exercise and Diet were both expressions of caring for the Body. And Spirituality was the overarching connection to something greater—the Spirit dimension that gave context and meaning to everything else.

But here's what became revolutionary in my understanding: these three dimensions aren't separate. They're more like three faces of a single crystal, each reflecting and influencing the others. A thought in the Mind creates chemistry in the Body. The state of the Body influences the clarity of the Mind. The Spirit dimension infuses both with purpose and connection to the greater whole.

MIND: THE CONTROL CENTER

The Mind dimension encompasses our thoughts, beliefs, emotions, and the stories we tell ourselves about our lives. It's the interpreter of experience, the meaning-maker, the part of us that can choose our response to any situation.

What I discovered was that the Mind isn't just along for the ride in healing—it's often driving the bus. Our thoughts create our biochemistry. Fear floods the body with cortisol stress hormones that suppress immune function. Hope and joy trigger cascades of healing hormones like dopamine, serotonin, and oxytocin. The placebo effect isn't a trick; it's proof of the Mind's power to influence physical reality.

BODY: THE SACRED VESSEL

The Body dimension is our physical form—not just muscles and organs, but the miraculous collection of 37 trillion cells working in concert. It's our interface with the physical world, the vessel through which we experience life.

I learned to see my body not as something that had betrayed me with cancer, but as an incredibly intelligent system that had been sending me messages I'd ignored. The tumor wasn't an enemy attack; it was the body's attempt to contain and isolate dysfunctional cells. My body hadn't failed—it had been crying for help while I was too busy to listen.

SPIRIT: THE ETERNAL ESSENCE

The Spirit dimension is perhaps the most difficult to define because it transcends definition. It's our connection to something greater than our individual self—whether you call it consciousness, soul, life force, or divine essence. It's what remains constant while everything else changes.

For me, connecting with Spirit meant recognizing that I am more than this temporary physical form and its accompanying thoughts. There's an awareness, a presence, that has been with me since my earliest memories and will continue beyond this body's expiration date. This wasn't just a comforting belief—it was a felt experience that arose in deep meditation.

THE INTEGRATION

Once I understood these three dimensions, my entire approach to healing transformed. Instead of doing meditation, exercise, diet, and sleep practices as separate activities, I began to see how each practice could consciously engage all three dimensions simultaneously.

When I meditated, I wasn't just calming my Mind—I was also sending healing signals to my Body and connecting with Spirit. When I exercised, I wasn't just moving my Body—I was also training my Mind in discipline and expressing gratitude through Spirit. When I ate, I wasn't just feeding my Body—I was making a mindful choice (Mind) and honoring the sacred act of nourishment (Spirit).

This integration created a multiplier effect. Each practice became more powerful because it was consciously engaging multiple dimensions of healing. The whole became exponentially greater than the sum of its parts.

CHAPTER 16:
HEALING THE MIND

The mind is everything. What you think you become.
— **Buddha**

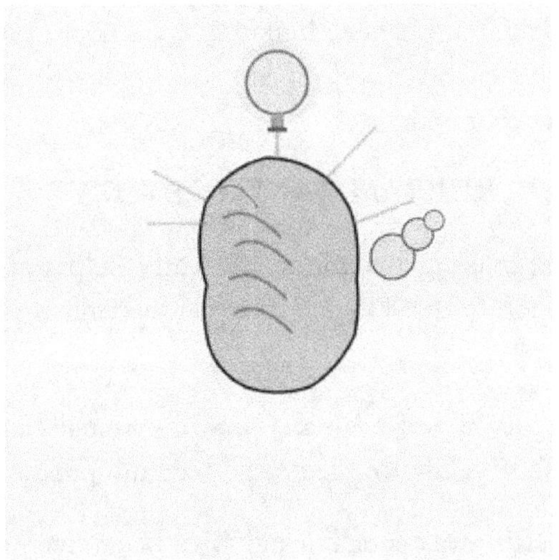

The mind is not your enemy, though it can feel that way during serious illness. When I was first diagnosed and as the fear of uncertainty took hold, my mind became a factory of worst-case scenarios, churning out fear, doubt, and despair with industrial efficiency. Every physical sensation became a sign of cancer spreading. Every statistic became my probable future. The mind that had served me so well in business and life had turned into a torture device.

But I learned something crucial: the mind is not fixed. It's plastic, moldable, trainable. The thoughts that seem so solid and real are actually just patterns—and patterns can be changed.

BECOMING THE OBSERVER

The first breakthrough came when I learned to observe my thoughts rather than be consumed by them. Through meditation, I discovered there's a part of me that can watch thoughts arise and pass without being swept away. This observer self became my refuge.

When fear arose—"What if the cancer comes back?"—I learned to notice it as just a thought, not a prophecy. I would acknowledge it: "I see you, fear. Thank you for trying to protect me. But I choose to focus on healing right now."

This wasn't denial or positive thinking. It was conscious choice about where to direct my mental energy. Fear would still visit, but it no longer moved in and redecorated.

REFRAMING THE STORY

We are meaning-making machines. We can't help but create stories about what happens to us. The key insight was realizing I could choose which story to tell.

The victim story was available: "I have terminal cancer. My life is over. This is unfair." This story led to despair and paralysis.

But another story was equally true: "I've been given a wake-up call. This is an opportunity to transform. I'm becoming who I was meant to be." This story led to empowerment and action.

Same facts, different frame. The facts didn't change—I had cancer. But how I related to those facts made all the difference. I chose the story that supported healing.

It's not the event that matters; it's the meaning we assign to the event that matters.

THE POWER OF MENTAL REHEARSAL

Athletes have long known that mental rehearsal improves performance. The brain doesn't fully distinguish between vividly imagined experience and real experience. I decided to use this for healing.

Every morning during meditation, I would spend time visualizing my body in perfect health. I would see my immune system as powerful and intelligent. I would imagine the areas where tumors had been now filled with healthy, vibrant tissue. I would feel the emotions of being completely healed—the joy, the gratitude, the freedom.

This wasn't wishful thinking. Studies show that visualization can influence immune function, reduce inflammation, and even affect gene expression. I was literally using my mind to reprogram my body.

EMOTIONAL ALCHEMY

Emotions are more than feelings—they're chemical events in the body. Anger releases different hormones than gratitude. Fear creates different proteins than love. I realized that managing my emotional state was as important as managing my diet.

But emotions can't just be suppressed or ignored. They need to be felt, acknowledged, and then consciously transformed. When anger arose about my diagnosis, I would feel it fully, then ask: "What is this anger protecting? What does it need?" Often, anger was just fear in disguise, and fear was just love with nowhere to go.

I developed what I called emotional alchemy—transforming lower emotions into higher ones:

1. Fear into curiosity: "What can this teach me?"

2. Anger into determination: "How can I channel this energy?"

3. Sadness into compassion: "How can this soften my heart?"

4. Despair into surrender: "What wants to emerge through this?"

STRESS AS THE SILENT KILLER

If I had to identify one factor that contributed most to my illness, it would be chronic stress. Not dramatic stress, but the constant, low-grade pressure of running a business, meeting expectations, and never quite relaxing. In retrospect, my unshakeable confidence—my belief that I could handle any challenge, no matter how difficult—created a hidden burden. I never acknowledged the toll it was taking. The stress wasn't obvious on the surface, but it was silently brewing beneath it.

Stress isn't just uncomfortable—it's literally toxic. Chronic stress suppresses immune function, increases inflammation, disrupts sleep, and creates an internal environment where disease thrives. Learning to manage stress wasn't optional for healing; it was essential.

I developed a toolkit for stress reduction:

1. **Breath work:** Four counts in, hold for four, four counts out. This activated my parasympathetic nervous system within minutes.

24. **Progressive relaxation:** Systematically tensing and releasing each muscle group.

25. **Mindfulness anchors:** Throughout the day, taking 30-second breaks to fully arrive in the present moment.

26. **Boundary setting:** Learning to say no to commitments that drained my energy.

Allowing enough time to perform a task. For example, I would allow an extra 15 minutes to take a trip to see the doctor and not get stressed because I am late for the appointment.

THE MIND-BODY FEEDBACK LOOP

Perhaps the most important discovery was understanding the constant conversation between mind and body. Every thought creates a chemical cascade. Every emotion triggers a physical response. But it works both ways—the state of the body influences the mind.

When I felt mentally stuck or emotionally heavy, I would change my physiology. Stand tall, breathe deep, smile (even if I didn't feel like it), move my body. The physical shift would create a mental shift. The body would teach the mind how to feel better.

This bi-directional influence became a powerful tool. I wasn't at the mercy of my thoughts or my body. I could intervene at either level to influence the whole system toward healing.

CHAPTER 17: HONORING THE BODY

Your body is precious. It is our vehicle for awakening.
Treat it with care.
— Buddha

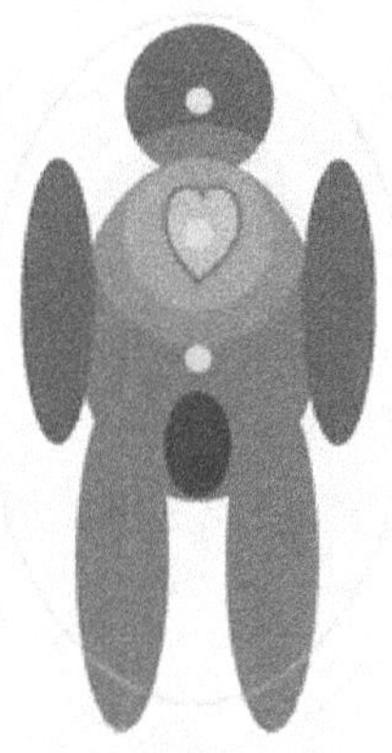

For most of my adult life, I treated my body like a rental car—using it hard, maintaining it minimally, assuming it would just keep running. I fed it whatever was convenient, slept when exhausted, and exercised sporadically. My body was simply the vehicle that carried my ambitious mind through life.

Cancer changed that relationship entirely. Suddenly, my body wasn't just transportation—it was the battlefield where my life was being decided. Every cell, every organ, every system needed to be recruited as an ally in healing. I had to learn to honor this physical form that I had taken for granted for so long.

THE BODY'S WISDOM

The first shift was recognizing that my body wasn't broken—it was incredibly intelligent. Cancer wasn't a malfunction; it was my body's response to conditions I had created through lifestyle, stress, and neglect. The tumor was the body's attempt to contain dysfunction, like building a wall around danger.

This perspective changed everything. Instead of seeing my body as the enemy that had betrayed me, I saw it as a wise teacher showing me what needed to change. Every symptom was communication. Every sensation was feedback. I just needed to learn the language.

THE HOLISTIC VIEW

Western medicine tends to compartmentalize the body—the oncologist treats cancer, the cardiologist treats the heart, the neurologist treats the brain. But the body doesn't work in departments. It's one integrated system where everything affects everything else.

I learned that gut health affects brain function through the vagus nerve. Inflammation in one area creates systemic effects. Hormonal imbalances influence immune function. Sleep quality impacts every single cellular process. The body is a symphony, not a collection of solo instruments.

This holistic understanding meant that healing couldn't be targeted at just the tumor site. I needed to create conditions for whole-body wellness, trusting that healthy systems would naturally address dysfunction.

SLEEP: THE ULTIMATE SUPERPOWER

If I could give cancer patients only one piece of advice, it would be this: protect your sleep as if your life depends on it—because it does.

I've dedicated Chapter 14 to the science and practice of healing sleep, so I won't repeat the details here. But in the context of honoring the body, I want to emphasize that sleep became the foundation upon which all other healing occurred. The sleep protocols I developed—creating a sleep sanctuary, becoming militant about sleep hygiene, and using guided meditations—became non-negotiable practices that supported every other aspect of my recovery.

THE HEALING ENVIRONMENT

I realized that healing doesn't happen in isolation—it happens in an environment. And I needed to create an environment that supported healing at every level.

This meant examining everything in my physical space:

Air quality: I invested in air purifiers and brought in plants that clean the air naturally.

Water: I installed filters to remove chlorine, fluoride, and other chemicals.

Light: I maximized natural sunlight during the day and used warm, dim lighting in the evening.

Sound: I reduced noise pollution and played healing frequencies and nature sounds.

Toxins: I eliminated chemical cleaners, synthetic fragrances, and plastic containers.

Nature: I spent time outdoors daily, grounding myself by walking barefoot on grass.

THE LYMPHATIC SYSTEM: THE FORGOTTEN HEALER

One of the most important discoveries in my healing journey was understanding the lymphatic system—the body's waste removal and immune transport network. Unlike the circulatory system, lymph doesn't have a pump. It relies entirely on movement and breathing to function.

During treatment, when I was sedentary, my lymph system became stagnant. Toxins accumulated, immune cells couldn't circulate efficiently, and healing slowed. I had to consciously activate this system:

Light stretching or yoga

Gentle resistance exercises

Dry brushing—stimulates lymph flow through the skin

Deep breathing—the diaphragm acts as a lymphatic pump

Yoga twists—compress and release lymph nodes

Hydration—lymph is mostly water and needs adequate fluid to flow

LISTENING TO THE BODY'S SIGNALS

Perhaps the most profound shift was learning to listen—really listen—to my body's signals. For years, I had overridden these signals with caffeine, painkillers, and sheer willpower. Now I realized these signals were my body's attempt to communicate its needs.

Fatigue meant rest, not push through. Hunger meant nourishment, not just filling the stomach. Pain meant attention needed, not suppression. Anxiety meant something was out of balance, not that I needed to work harder.

I developed a practice of body scanning—regularly checking in with each part of my body, asking what it needed, and actually responding to those needs. This wasn't indulgence; it was intelligent cooperation with the 37 trillion cells working to keep me alive.

The body, I learned, is not just a physical machine. It's a conscious, intelligent system that wants to thrive. When we honor it—truly honor it—with proper nutrition, movement, rest, and attention, it responds with vitality and healing beyond what we thought possible.

CHAPTER 18:
AWAKENING THE SPIRIT

The soul always knows what to do to heal itself. The challenge is to silence the mind.
— **Caroline Myss**

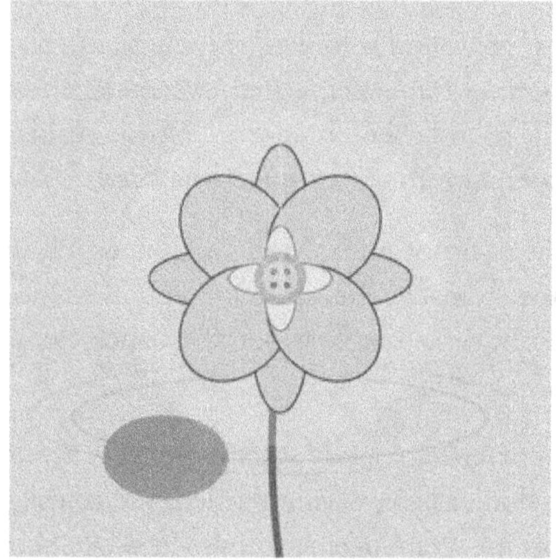

Of the three dimensions—Mind, Body, and Spirit—Spirit was simultaneously the most important and the most elusive. It couldn't be measured in lab tests or seen on scans. There was no scientific protocol for spiritual healing. Yet I came to understand that without addressing the spiritual dimension, all other healing efforts were incomplete.

Spirit isn't about religion, though religion can be one path to it. Spirit is about connection—to something greater than our individual self, to the essence of who we are beyond our temporary physical form, to the infinite intelligence that orchestrates life itself.

BEYOND THE PHYSICAL SELF

The cancer diagnosis forced me to confront a fundamental question: Who am I, really? If my body was failing, if my cognitive abilities were compromised by chemo brain, if my roles as entrepreneur and provider were stripped away—what remained?

Through meditation and contemplation, I discovered something profound. Behind all the changing aspects of my life—my body, thoughts, emotions, roles—there was something unchanging. A presence, an awareness, that had been with me since my earliest memories. This awareness wasn't affected by cancer. It wasn't diminished by treatment. It simply was.

This recognition was liberating. If my essential nature transcended the physical, then even death lost its ultimate sting. Yes, this body would eventually cease, but the essence of who I am—consciousness itself—felt eternal, or at least independent of physical form.

THE FEAR OF DEATH TRANSFORMED

Before cancer, I rarely thought about death. It was an abstract concept, something that happened to other people, older people, unlucky people. Cancer eliminated that comfortable distance. Death became a real possibility, perhaps a probability, certainly an inevitability.

The fear was primal and overwhelming at first. Not just fear of pain or the unknown, but fear of non-existence, of everything I am simply ceasing. This fear created constant background anxiety that poisoned every moment.

But as I explored the spiritual dimension, the fear began to transform. Through deep meditation, I experienced states where 'I' seemed to disappear, yet awareness remained. If awareness could exist without my usual sense of self, perhaps death was not the extinction I feared but a transition to a different form of existence.

I studied near-death experiences, finding remarkable consistency in reports of expanded consciousness, profound peace, and connection to infinite love. Whether these were real glimpses beyond the veil or the brain's way of easing transition didn't matter. They pointed to possibilities beyond material existence.

LETTING GO

The spiritual journey required letting go of everything I thought I knew about how life should unfold. My plans, my timeline, my need to control outcomes—all had to be released.

This wasn't giving up or becoming passive. It was recognizing that my small, ego-driven will was not the only force at play. There was a larger intelligence, a flow to life that I could either resist or align with. Resistance created suffering. Alignment created peace.

I learned to hold my desires lightly—yes, I wanted to heal, to live, to see my grandchildren. But I held these wants with open hands, not clenched fists. If life had other plans, I would meet them with as much grace as possible.

GRATITUDE AS SPIRITUAL PRACTICE

Gratitude became my primary spiritual practice. Not gratitude for cancer—I'm not that evolved—but gratitude for everything cancer revealed: the love of my family, the preciousness of each day, the strength I didn't know I had, the spiritual dimensions I might never have explored.

Each morning, I would list ten things I was grateful for, feeling the emotion of appreciation, not just thinking the thoughts. This wasn't toxic positivity or denial of difficulty. It was conscious redirection of attention from lack to abundance, from fear to love.

Gratitude literally changed my biochemistry. Studies show it increases dopamine and serotonin, reduces inflammatory markers, and strengthens immune function. But beyond the science, gratitude connected me to the sacred dimension of ordinary life. A glass of water became a miracle. A bird's song became a symphony. My wife's smile became a glimpse of the divine.

FINDING MEANING IN SUFFERING

Perhaps the most profound spiritual question was: What is the meaning of this suffering? Why cancer? Why me? Why now?

I never found a satisfactory intellectual answer. But I found something better—a felt sense that this experience, as difficult as it was, was somehow necessary for my evolution. Not punishment, not random misfortune, but a catalyst for transformation I couldn't have achieved any other way.

Cancer cracked me open. It shattered my ego's illusion of control. It forced me to face my mortality, examine my priorities, and discover dimensions of existence I had ignored. In a strange way I'm still uncomfortable admitting, cancer gave me gifts I didn't know I needed.

CONNECTION TO THE INFINITE

The deepest spiritual experiences came in meditation when the boundaries of self dissolved. In these moments, there was no cancer patient, no separate self struggling to heal. There was just consciousness, vast and peaceful, connected to everything and nothing.

These experiences weren't hallucinations or wishful thinking. They were more real than ordinary reality, though impossible to fully convey in words. They showed me that what I truly am is not limited to this body-mind that will inevitably pass away. There's something eternal, infinite, and perfect at the core of being.

This connection to the infinite became my ultimate medicine. Not because it cured cancer—that's not how spirituality works—but because it cured my deepest fear: the fear that I am separate, alone, and temporary. When that fear dissolved, everything else became workable.

LIVING AS SPIRIT

The spiritual dimension isn't separate from daily life—it infuses everything when we're aware of it. Washing dishes becomes a meditation. Walking becomes a prayer. Breathing becomes communion with life itself.

I learned to see every person as a spiritual being having a human experience, just like me. The checkout clerk, the nurse, the fellow patient—all expressions of the same consciousness wearing different masks. This recognition created instant connection and dissolved the isolation that illness can bring.

THE COMPLETE TRINITY

With all three dimensions—Mind, Body, and Spirit—consciously engaged, healing became something greater than just eliminating disease. It became a return to wholeness, an integration of all aspects of being.

The Mind provided focus and direction. The Body provided the vessel for transformation. The Spirit provided meaning and connection to something greater. Together, they created a healing synergy that no single approach could achieve.

This wasn't just about surviving cancer. It was about discovering who I really am and living from that truth. In that sense, the healing had already occurred, regardless of what the scans would show. I was whole, not because my body was perfect, but because I had reconnected with the perfection that was always there, waiting to be recognized.

The evolution from MEDS to Mind-Body-Spirit wasn't just a change in framework—it was a fundamental shift in how I understood healing, health, and what it means to be truly alive. This understanding would guide not just my recovery, but the entire remainder of my life, however long that might be.

PART *Six*

THE DEEPER WORK

Integration and Transformation

CHAPTER 19:
HEALING HIDDEN WOUNDS

The privilege of a lifetime is to become who you truly are.
— **Carl Jung**

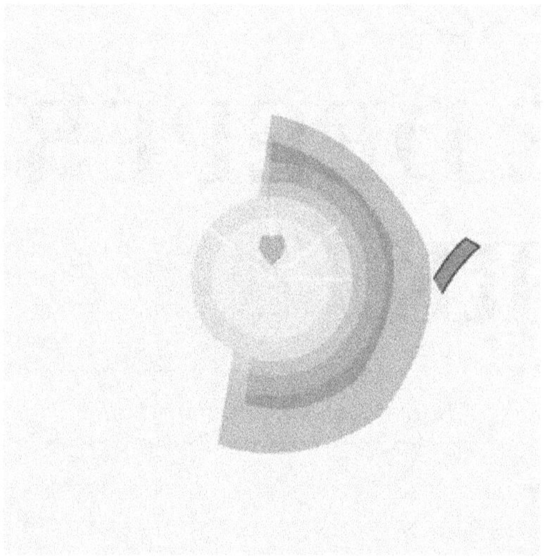

The relentless progression of disease had forced me into a profound confrontation. Each hurdle brought its share of pain, fear, and uncertainty, but what surprised me most was how these external challenges forced an internal reckoning. Physical healing, I discovered, could not be separated from emotional and psychological healing. To truly heal, I had to address wounds I didn't even know existed.

EMOTIONAL RESILIENCE IN THE FACE OF PAIN

Physical illness is rarely just physical. Disease flourishes in the presence of unresolved emotional trauma, chronic stress, and deep-seated negative patterns. My healing journey required me to look beneath the surface of my symptoms and confront the emotional landscape I had long ignored.

The entrepreneurial drive that had served me so well in business had also created a pattern of chronic stress. I had been running on adrenaline for decades, pushing through exhaustion, ignoring my body's signals, prioritizing achievement over wellbeing. My nervous system had been locked in fight-or-flight mode for so long that I didn't even remember what true relaxation felt like.

Cancer forced me to stop. Not just slow down, but truly stop. In that stillness, emotions I had suppressed for years began to surface. Anger I hadn't acknowledged. Grief I hadn't processed. Fears I had buried under layers of competence and confidence.

ACKNOWLEDGING GRIEF

One of the most profound realizations was the depth of grief I carried. Not just grief about the cancer diagnosis, but older griefs I had never fully processed. The loss of my identity as a healthy, invincible person. The loss of my carefree relationship with my body. The loss of certainty about my future.

But there were older griefs too. Disappointments from my past. Dreams that hadn't materialized. Relationships that had ended. Parts of myself I had abandoned in the pursuit of success. All of this unprocessed grief had been stored in my body, creating an emotional toxicity that paralleled the physical disease.

I learned that grief unexpressed becomes grief embodied. The body holds what the mind won't process. Through therapy, journaling, and meditation, I gave voice to these buried sorrows. I cried tears that were decades overdue, saying everything I wished I had said, allowing myself to fully feel the weight of what had been lost.

This is not wallowing or self-pity. It is necessary cleansing. Each tear released, each emotion acknowledged, created more space for healing.

The energy that had been used to suppress these feelings became available for recovery.

RECONSTRUCTING IDENTITY

Perhaps the most challenging aspect was reconstructing my identity. For so long, I had defined myself by my achievements, my roles, my capabilities. I was the successful entrepreneur. The provider. The problem-solver. The one others turned to for strength.

Cancer stripped away these external identities. I couldn't work at my previous pace. I couldn't provide in the same way. I couldn't be the strong one when I was barely holding on myself. Who was I without these roles?

This identity crisis was terrifying but ultimately liberating. I discovered that beneath all the roles and achievements was something simpler and truer: I was a human being worthy of love and belonging simply because I existed, not because of what I could do or provide.

I began to build a new identity based not on doing but on being. I was a consciousness experiencing life. I was a soul on a journey. I was love expressing itself through a temporary physical form. These identities couldn't be threatened by illness or loss of function. They were unchangeable, eternal aspects of who I truly am.

THE POWER OF FORGIVENESS

As I excavated these emotional layers, I discovered pockets of resentment and blame I didn't know existed. Resentment toward people who had hurt me. Blame toward myself for choices I had made. Anger at life for dealing me this hand.

These resentments were like emotional tumors, poisoning my system from within. I realized that forgiveness wasn't optional for healing—it was essential. But forgiveness didn't mean condoning harmful behavior or pretending things were okay when they weren't. Forgiveness meant releasing the emotional charge, freeing myself from the prison of past pain.

I started with forgiving myself. For the years of self-neglect. For ignoring my body's signals. For the stress I had created through my choices. For not being perfect. This self-forgiveness was perhaps the hardest but most important step.

Then I moved to forgiving others. Not in person—many of these people were no longer in my life. But in my heart, I released them. I visualized cutting energetic cords that bound me to past pain.

Finally, I had to forgive life itself. Forgive the unfairness of disease. Forgive the randomness of suffering. Forgive God or the universe or whatever force had allowed this to happen. This wasn't about understanding why—I may never understand why. It was about releasing the resistance and accepting what is.

RELATIONSHIPS AND INTIMACY: NAVIGATING LOVE THROUGH ILLNESS

Cancer doesn't just affect the patient—it transforms every relationship. My wife became my caregiver as well as my partner. My children became witnesses to my vulnerability. Friends didn't know how to act around me. Some relationships deepened while others fell away.

The most profound impact was on my marriage. My wife and I had been partners for decades, but cancer introduced dynamics we had never navigated. She had to watch me suffer without being able to fix it. I had to accept help with tasks I had always handled myself. We both had to face the possibility of my death and what that would mean for her future.

We had to learn new ways of communicating. I had to express needs I had never voiced before. She had to share fears and anger she had been hiding to protect me. We had to be more honest than ever before, because time felt too precious to waste on pretense.

SETTING BOUNDARIES

One unexpected aspect of emotional healing was learning to set boundaries. For years, I had been available to everyone—employees, friends, extended family. I prided myself on being helpful, reliable, always there when needed. But this pattern had contributed to my depletion.

Cancer gave me permission to say no. No to commitments that drained me. No to relationships that were meaningless. No to obligations that didn't align with my healing. This wasn't selfishness—it was survival.

Some people understood and respected these boundaries. Others were offended or disappeared from my life. This natural selection of relationships was painful but necessary. I learned that the people who truly cared for me wanted what was best for my healing, even if it meant I was less available to them.

THE SHADOW WORK

Perhaps the deepest emotional work involved confronting what Jung called the shadow—the parts of myself I had rejected or hidden. The weakness I had never wanted to show. The neediness I had always denied. The fear I had covered with bravado. The vulnerability I had armored against.

Cancer brought all of these shadow aspects into the light. I couldn't pretend to be strong when I could barely walk. I couldn't deny neediness when I required help with basic tasks. I couldn't hide fear when mortality was knocking at my door.

At first, this exposure felt like death—the death of the false self I had constructed. But as I learned to accept these shadow aspects, to even embrace them, something remarkable happened. They became sources of strength. My vulnerability allowed others to connect with me more deeply. My neediness taught me to receive love. My fear became a gateway to courage.

EMOTIONAL HEALING AS PHYSICAL MEDICINE

What amazed me most was how this emotional work translated into physical healing. As I released old grief, my body felt lighter. As I forgave, inflammation decreased. As I set boundaries, my energy increased. As I embraced my shadow, my immune system seemed to strengthen.

This wasn't just my imagination. Research in psychoneuroimmunology shows clear connections between emotional states and immune function. Chronic negative emotions suppress immune activity. Positive emotions enhance it. By healing emotionally, I was literally changing my body's ability to heal physically.

The hidden wounds—those emotional and psychological injuries I had carried for years—turned out to be as important to address as the tumor itself. Perhaps more so, because while the tumor could be removed surgically, these emotional wounds would continue generating disease-promoting stress until they were healed.

This deeper work wasn't easy. It required courage to face what I had spent decades avoiding. It required vulnerability to admit my wounds. It required persistence to keep going when the process was painful. But it was essential. True healing, I learned, happens from the inside out, starting with the hidden wounds we carry in our hearts.

CHAPTER 20:
LESSONS FROM THE JOURNEY

We are not human beings having a spiritual experience. We are spiritual beings having a human experience.
— Pierre Teilhard de Chardin

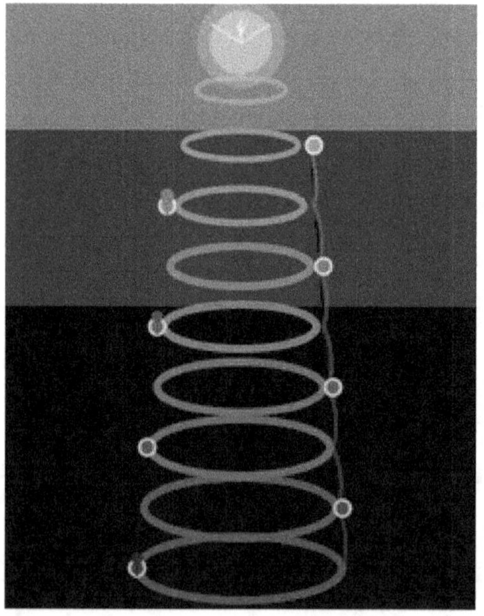

If someone had told me six years ago that cancer would become one of my greatest teachers, I would have thought them insane. Who wants a teacher that threatens your life, disrupts everything you've built, and forces you to confront your deepest fears? Yet here I am, grateful for lessons I could have learned in no other way.

These lessons didn't come all at once. They arrived the way seasons change—imperceptibly at first, then undeniably. Each phase of the journey—diagnosis, treatment, recovery, integration—offered its own wisdom. Now, with the benefit of perspective, I can see the complete picture of what this experience has taught me.

THE POWER OF CHOICE IN EVERY MOMENT

Perhaps the most fundamental lesson was discovering that even when we can't control what happens to us, we always have choice in how we respond. Viktor Frankl, a Holocaust survivor, called this "the last of human freedoms"—the ability to choose one's attitude in any given circumstance.

Cancer took away many choices. I couldn't choose not to have it. I couldn't choose to skip the suffering. I couldn't choose guaranteed healing. But within these constraints, countless choices remained. I could choose hope over despair. I could choose to see opportunity in crisis. I could choose to focus on what I could control rather than lamenting what I couldn't.

This power of choice extended to the smallest moments. When nausea struck, I could choose to resist and amplify the discomfort, or breathe and let it pass through me. When fear arose, I could choose to spiral into worst-case scenarios, or acknowledge the fear and return to the present. When faced with statistical prognoses, I could choose to accept them as my fate, or see them as averages that didn't determine my individual outcome.

Each choice, no matter how small, was a declaration of agency. In a situation where so much felt out of control, these choices became my way of maintaining dignity, hope, and active participation in my healing.

REFRAMING ADVERSITY AS A TEACHER

The mind's tendency is to label cancer as "bad," "enemy," "disaster." This labeling creates resistance, and resistance creates suffering. One of the most powerful shifts was learning to reframe cancer not as an enemy to defeat but as a teacher with difficult lessons.

What if cancer wasn't trying to kill me but trying to wake me up? What if it was showing me all the ways I had been slowly killing myself through stress, neglect, and disconnection from what truly mattered? What if this crisis was actually an opportunity for transformation I wouldn't have chosen but desperately needed?

This reframe didn't make cancer good or desirable. I wouldn't wish this experience on anyone. But it transformed my relationship with the disease from antagonistic to curious. Instead of "Why is this happening to me?" I began asking "What is this here to teach me?"

The lessons were profound: slow down, listen to your body, prioritize what matters, express love freely, release what you cannot control, find meaning in difficulty, and discover strength you didn't know existed.

THE IMPORTANCE OF MINDSET IN HEALING

Through this journey, I became convinced that mindset isn't just important for healing—it's foundational. Two patients with identical diagnoses and treatments can have vastly different outcomes, and often the difference is mindset.

This isn't about fake positivity or denying the seriousness of disease. It's about choosing thoughts that support rather than sabotage healing. The patient who believes they will die often does. The patient who believes they will heal has a fighting chance. The mind's beliefs become the body's biology.

I witnessed this in treatment centers. Patients who saw themselves as victims, who had given up hope, who constantly spoke of their illness, seemed to decline rapidly. Those who maintained hope, who focused on reasons to live, who saw themselves as temporarily dealing with disease rather than being defined by it, often exceeded medical expectations.

I chose to cultivate what I call a "healing mindset":

1. Expecting positive outcomes while accepting whatever comes

2. Focusing on progress, not perfection

3. Celebrating small victories

4. Speaking of healing, not illness

5. Visualizing desired outcomes

6. Maintaining gratitude even in difficulty

SUPPORT SYSTEMS: YOU CANNOT HEAL ALONE

As an entrepreneur, I was accustomed to solving problems myself. Independence was a source of pride. Cancer shattered this illusion of self-sufficiency. I learned that healing requires community, support, and the humility to receive help.

My wife became my anchor, providing not just practical support but emotional stability when I was falling apart. My children showed up in ways that revealed their depth and maturity. Friends who truly cared made themselves known through consistent presence, while fair-weather relationships naturally fell away.

But support came from unexpected sources too. The nurse who took care of me all night after a particularly difficult bladder surgery and treatment. The fellow patient who shared their story of hope. The stranger who smiled at me when I was waiting for radiation therapy and obviously ill, seeing me as a person, not a disease.

I learned to receive—truly receive—help without feeling diminished. To say "yes" when someone offered assistance. To admit when I was struggling. To let others care for me without feeling I had to immediately reciprocate. This receiving was its own form of healing, teaching me that vulnerability creates connection and that we're all interconnected in ways we rarely acknowledge.

LISTENING TO THE BODY'S INTELLIGENCE

Before cancer, I treated my body like a machine—pushing it when tired, medicating it when sick, ignoring its signals when inconvenient. Cancer taught me that the body has its own intelligence, constantly communicating through sensations, symptoms, and subtle signals.

I learned to distinguish between different types of fatigue—the healing fatigue that required rest versus the deconditioning fatigue that needed gentle movement. I learned to read my energy levels like a fuel gauge, planning activities when energy was highest and resting before hitting empty.

Pain became a teacher rather than an enemy. Sharp pain meant stop immediately. Dull ache meant proceed with caution. Absence of pain after prolonged pain meant healing was happening. Each sensation was information, guidance from my body about what it needed.

Most importantly, I learned to trust my body's wisdom over external protocols. When a recommended supplement made me feel worse, I stopped taking it despite the research supporting it. When my body craved certain foods, I honored those cravings (within reason). When conventional wisdom said push through, but my body said rest, I rested.

LIVING WITH UNCERTAINTY

Perhaps the most challenging lesson was learning to live with radical uncertainty. Before cancer, I lived under the illusion of control and predictability. I made five-year plans. I assumed linear progression. I expected that effort would equal outcome.

Cancer obliterated these illusions. I didn't know if I'd live six months or sixty years. Each scan brought the possibility of good news or devastating setback. Treatments might work or might fail. Side effects might be manageable or overwhelming. The future became completely unknowable.

At first, this uncertainty was paralyzing. How do you plan when you don't know if you'll be here? How do you hope when statistics suggest otherwise? How do you invest in a future that might not exist?

The answer came through a paradox: by fully accepting uncertainty, I found peace. I stopped needing to know the outcome. I stopped trying to control the uncontrollable. I learned to hold plans lightly, to hope without attachment, to invest fully in each day without requiring guarantees about tomorrow.

This acceptance of uncertainty extended beyond cancer. I realized that uncertainty had always been the truth—I just hadn't seen it. No one knows their expiration date. Control has always been an illusion. The future has never been guaranteed. Cancer just made these truths impossible to ignore.

THE PRACTICE OF PRESENCE

With the future uncertain and the past irrelevant to healing, I was left with only one temporal location: now. The present moment became not just a spiritual concept but a practical necessity.

When I projected into the future, anxiety arose. When I dwelt on the past, regret surfaced. But in the present moment, I was simply alive. Breathing. Existing. Usually okay, even in difficult circumstances.

This presence transformed ordinary moments into extraordinary ones. The warmth of sunlight through a window became something to feel grateful for. A shared meal became a sacred act. The simple fact of breathing—in and out, without effort—became astonishing.

I realized I had spent most of my life absent from my life—physically present but mentally elsewhere, planning, analyzing, worrying. Cancer brought me home to the only moment that exists: this one.

INTEGRATION: LIVING THE LESSONS FORWARD

These lessons weren't meant to be temporary adjustments during crisis. They were invitations to a different way of living. As I moved from active treatment to recovery to whatever comes next, the challenge became integrating these lessons into daily life.

It would be easy to slip back into old patterns as the crisis recedes. To forget the preciousness of time when death feels distant again. To stop listening to my body when it's not screaming. To abandon presence for productivity.

But these lessons came at too high a price to abandon. They're not just concepts I learned but truths I lived. They're encoded in my cells, written in my scars, embedded in my transformed identity.

Living these lessons forward means making different choices. Prioritizing being over doing. Choosing presence over productivity. Maintaining boundaries that protect my energy. Continuing practices that nourish body, mind, and spirit. Remembering that each day is a gift, not a guarantee.

The journey continues, and new lessons emerge. But these foundational teachings from the cancer journey have become my compass, guiding me toward a life that's not just longer but deeper, not just survived but truly lived.

MOMENTS THAT MATTERED

Life is not measured by the number of breaths we take, but by the moments that take our breath away.
— **Maya Angelou**

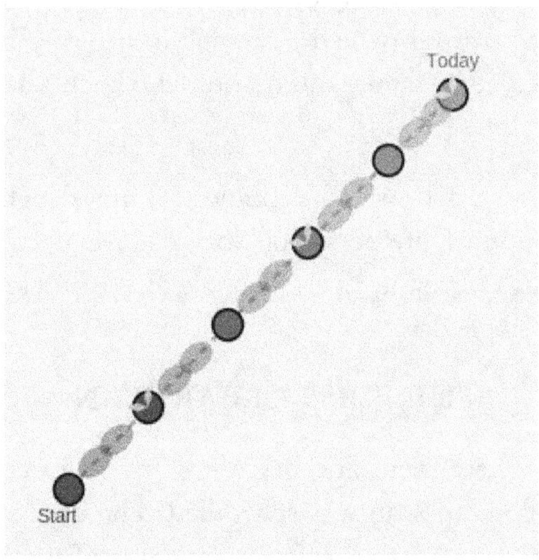

Life is not measured in years but in moments. Cancer taught me this truth with crystal clarity. When facing mortality, time becomes less about quantity and more about quality. Looking back on my journey, it's not the treatments or protocols I remember most vividly—it's specific moments that defined the experience and transformed me.

THE DAUGHTER'S WEDDING: A MILESTONE OF LOVE

When I was diagnosed in June, my daughter's wedding was just three months away. The doctors couldn't guarantee I'd make it. The treatment schedule would put me right in the middle of radiation during her big day. My greatest fear wasn't dying—it was missing this moment.

September came, and despite the fatigue, despite the ongoing treatment, I was there. Not just present, but fully present. Walking her down the aisle, I felt time slow down. Each step was deliberate, sacred. I noticed everything—the way sunlight filtered through the trees, the tears in her eyes mixing with joy, the weight of her arm in mine.

Inside I was saying: I lived to see this. Love conquered fear. This moment is worth everything I've endured.

After the vows, I hugged her and my daughter whispered, "I'm so glad you're here, Dad." Tears rolled down my face and I couldn't speak. I just held her closer, memorizing the moment—her dress rustling against my suit, the song playing (which I can still hear perfectly), the warmth of being surrounded by family and friends who knew what this moment meant.

That wedding wasn't just a celebration of my daughter's marriage. It was a celebration of life persisting, love enduring, and the power of having something to live for. Every struggle of the previous months was justified by that single day.

THE FIRST CLEAR SCAN

After completing treatment and beginning my holistic healing protocol, the first follow-up scan was scheduled. The days leading up to it were torture. "Scanxiety" they call it—the unique form of anxiety that comes before medical imaging that will determine your fate.

I tried to stay positive, but my mind conjured every scenario. What if it had spread? What if the natural approach wasn't working? What if this was it?

The day came. The MRI machine's loud clicking that had once terrified me now felt familiar. I meditated through the procedure, sending love to every cell in my body, visualizing clear results.

Three days later, my oncologist said on our video call. "The scan is clear," she said. "No sign of recurrence." I asked her to repeat it. Clear. The word rang like a bell in my consciousness.

My wife and kids were present on the call and we all could barely contain our excitement and joy. That moment validated every meditation, every dietary change, every supplement, every prayer. The path less traveled had led somewhere beautiful.

THE RETURN TO TABLE TENNIS

Table tennis was where this journey began—missing shots I should have made, my body signaling that something was wrong. For months after treatment, I couldn't even think about playing. The association was too painful, the physical demands too great.

But one day, three years after surgery, I felt the pull to return to the table. Not to compete—just to hit the ball. The surgery had removed the tumor from my occipital lobe, the region responsible for peripheral vision. I wanted to know: had my vision improved or worsened after three years?

I went to the Club with my wife during a quiet hour, stood at the table, and picked up the paddle. My hand trembled—not from weakness, but from emotion and the fear of the unknown.

The first few hits were awkward. My timing was off, my movements uncertain. But gradually, muscle memory returned. The rhythm came back slowly.

Then an old friend walked in—a very skilled player. I asked him to volley with me. It took a few minutes to adjust to his faster pace and spin, but I found my way back to a natural rhythm. After several minutes, I could maintain ten to twenty volleys without missing a return.

And then, one perfect shot: a difficult cross-table return that required precision and timing. I made it. That was the victory moment—proof that I hadn't lost everything.

I stood there, paddle in hand, realizing I had come full circle. The place where my body first warned me of danger had become the place where it celebrated recovery. That table, that simple game, held my entire journey—from symptom to diagnosis to treatment to healing.

THE CONVERSATION WITH MY SON

My son had been stoic throughout my illness. While my daughter expressed emotions freely, he held his inside, being strong, being practical, being there without drama. I knew he was struggling but didn't know how to reach him.

One evening, months into recovery, we were alone together walking in the neighborhood. Out of nowhere, the walls came down. We talked for hours—about fear, philosophy and mortality, what he had felt but couldn't say, what I had experienced but couldn't share.

That conversation healed something between us. The cancer experience had forced us both to confront emotions we would normally avoid. In sharing them, we moved from father-son to two men who had faced the possibility of loss and found their way to deeper connection.

THE SUNRISE MEDITATION

There was one morning, about six months after diagnosis, when I woke before dawn. Instead of trying to fall back asleep, I felt called to meditate. I went to our backyard, sat on a cushion, and closed my eyes as the world was still dark.

As I meditated, the sun began to rise. With my eyes closed, I could feel the gradual warming, see the light changing through my eyelids. When I finally opened my eyes, the world was transformed—golden light everywhere, birds singing, dew sparkling on grass.

In that moment, I felt completely aligned with life itself. The sunrise wasn't just happening around me—it was happening within me. I understood viscerally that I was not separate from nature but part of it. The same force that raised the sun was healing my cells. The same intelligence that orchestrated the dawn was orchestrating my recovery.

That sunrise meditation became a touchstone moment. Whenever I doubted my healing or felt disconnected from life force, I would remember that morning—the light, the warmth, the absolute certainty that I was held by something infinite and loving.

THE DAY I CHOSE TO LIVE

There was a specific day, during the worst of treatment, when I made a conscious choice to live. Not hope to live, not try to live, but choose to live. It was different from survival instinct. It was a deliberate decision.

I had been vomiting all night from chemo. I was exhausted beyond description. My body felt like it was failing. In that dark moment, a voice inside said, "You could let go. No one would blame you."

I sat with that possibility. The release it offered. The end of suffering. And then, from somewhere deeper, came another voice: "No. Not yet. There's more to do, more to experience, more to give."

In that moment, I chose. Not just to survive but to thrive. Not just to endure but to transform. Not just to exist but to live fully. That choice changed everything. It wasn't a one-time decision but one I had to remake daily, sometimes hourly. But that first conscious choice set the direction for everything that followed.

SMALL MOMENTS, PROFOUND IMPACT

Beyond these milestone moments were countless small ones that mattered just as much:

The morning I could taste food again after weeks of metallic chemo taste.

The first time I walked around the block without resting.

My wife sleeping in the hospital chair, refusing to leave my side.

A text from a friend saying simply, "Thinking of you."

Laughing—really laughing—for the first time after diagnosis.

Each of these moments was a small victory, a tiny resurrection, a reason to continue. They taught me that healing happens in moments, not months. Recovery is not a destination but a series of small returns to life.

THE ONGOING MOMENT

Perhaps the most important moment is the one happening right now. As I write this, as you read this, we are sharing a moment across time and space. My journey has led to this moment of connection, this opportunity to share what I've learned.

Every moment since diagnosis has been a gift. Not because cancer is a gift—I still wouldn't wish this on anyone. But because awareness of mortality makes each moment precious. The ordinary becomes extraordinary when you realize it might not last.

These moments that mattered weren't all pleasant. Some were agonizing. Some were terrifying. But they were all profound in their ability to teach, transform, and reveal what truly matters: love, presence, connection, and the mysterious resilience of the human spirit.

The moments continue to accumulate. Each clear scan. Each birthday celebrated. Each ordinary Tuesday that I'm alive to witness. They matter not because they're special, but because I'm here to experience them. That, perhaps, is the greatest lesson: every moment matters when you're truly present for it.

CHAPTER 22:
FAMILY PERSPECTIVES

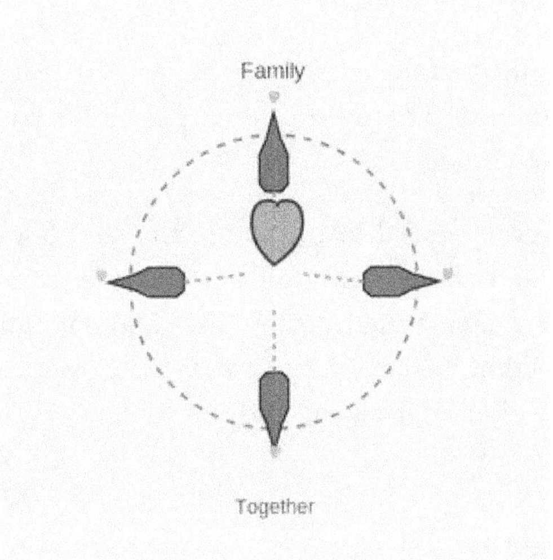

The journey of healing from cancer is never walked alone. While this book tells my story, my healing was deeply intertwined with my family's own journeys—their fears, their sacrifices, their transformations. I asked my wife Anu, my daughter Jaya, my son Ravi, and my son-in-law Vipul to share their perspectives. Their words reveal the hidden struggles I couldn't fully see at the time, and they complete the picture of what healing truly means—not just for the patient, but for the entire family ecosystem.

A WIFE'S JOURNEY THROUGH UNCERTAINTY—ANU'S PERSPECTIVE

The Day Everything Changed

Purna and I went in to see the doctor after his brain scan. We had no idea why she wanted us in her office for the results. She seemed so serious and sad when she told us Purna had brain cancer and it seemed slightly surreal. We both listened to her carefully and didn't really have many questions. She said that surgery was already being scheduled to remove the tumor. We both walked out not really knowing how to react. I don't recall feeling panic or strong emotions, only a kind of detached feeling of surprise.

Purna said in the parking lot, "Well, that was interesting... I guess we will have to figure out what to do next." I took his hand and said we would figure it out together.

Since the surgery needed to happen in the next few days, I put my emotions aside and started reaching out to all the major hospitals in the country that treated brain cancers. I had appointments for Purna at many of them within the next day or two. Luckily, we were able to connect with a great doctor at UCSF, and the surgery was scheduled right away.

Holding It Together

Purna was so cheerful and optimistic that it was hard to be down around him. We shared the news with the kids, and we finally had our emotional moment—tears and hugs around the kitchen table. I felt very supported by the kids and our soon-to-be son-in-law.

Purna did not want to share this news with anyone else, but I did tell my sister and another good friend. They both showed up at the hospital while he went through the surgery. It was then that fear finally hit me as we waited long hours. I remember walking out and going for a solitary walk in the park, feeling overwhelmed by grief and fear, feeling very alone and not wanting to break down in front of the kids.

Watching Him Change

After the surgery, Purna recovered quickly and then went through a very difficult chemo and radiation schedule. His cheerfulness slowly faded away as the treatment took its toll, but he still went to work every day and went to the gym every day. Perhaps that created an environment and feeling that everything is normal even though we knew it was not. As I saw his body become weaker, I experienced many emotions seeing the strong man I knew now becoming so frail. It was very difficult to see that and not be affected.

His only desire was to make it to our daughter's wedding. I did not have the luxury of indulging my emotions, as both the treatment and the wedding planning were going on at the same time. Most of the people in our life did not know what Purna was going through, so it was sometimes hard to be cheerful when meeting friends and family.

The Second Blow

When Purna got the bladder cancer diagnosis, it felt like too much. I remember saying to the Universe, "Really, another hit—you are not done yet?" Purna, however, said it's okay—we can handle it.

The bladder cancer treatment was even harder. I remember sitting on the sofa with Purna and weeping at the pain and suffering he was enduring. It was the low point in the entire experience. I think he also was deeply affected by the physical suffering and wondering if it was all worth it.

A Different Path

When Purna refused all further treatments for brain cancer, it was a difficult pill to swallow. I did not want to lose him, but I also could not see him suffering. Life without him would be difficult to imagine. We had been together for over four decades, and I had found my best friend in him. I was angry for some time but finally gave in when I saw that he could not be dissuaded. He was following his own path for healing, and I agreed to help him in that. The kids were also very upset, but nothing could change Purna's mind.

The Spiritual Awakening

Purna was very upbeat all the time and always felt that death is a part of life and not to be feared. We would try our best to heal the cancer, but whatever the outcome was, it was okay with him. He was at peace.

I remember being very upset one day and telling him I did not want him to die. He asked me, "Anu, how many years will be enough for you? Another 5 years, 10 years?" That really landed. I realized that either my time with him was enough right now, or it would never be enough.

It was then that cancer became a spiritual journey for me and, I think, our entire family. It taught me to let go of my illusion of control over life. It taught me to value every moment of a normal day and not look ahead. I re-engaged with the things that brought joy and happiness into our lives and made sure we did something every day that brought that feeling to life.

Milestones and Miracles

Our daughter's wedding was a very emotional experience for the entire family. I was so happy to see her getting married to a wonderful man, and yet at the same time, there were moments of sharp grief that Purna would not be around to see his grandkids and that we would not grow old together. Jaya's wedding vows talked about some of the challenges our family had gone through, and it brought tears and love at the same time.

Even though Purna was very much at peace, he did go through a few weeks of having nightmares. I'm sure he was coming to terms with his own fears.

Purna had brain scans every few months to monitor the cancer. It was very stressful as we waited for the results every time. Then the great relief that he had dodged the cancer for another few months. As the results kept coming back as stable, the stress slowly faded over time.

Transformation Through Trial

Purna has become my spiritual mentor as well as my best friend. I have learned how to navigate life gracefully by watching him go through something very difficult with humor and optimism and great surrender. I hope we grow old and grey together, surrounded by kids and grandchildren and family and friends.

There have been many wonderful moments in the last few years since his diagnosis. Jaya getting married and our first grandchild being born. Our life is full and lacks nothing. I know now that you only have today. Nothing else is guaranteed, and it is enough.

A DAUGHTER'S JOURNEY FROM FEAR TO ACCEPTANCE — JAYA'S PERSPECTIVE

I still remember that night very vividly—Ravi and I drove down to Fremont late on a Friday, tired, with a bad headache, just wanting to get home. We settled into the living room the way we always did. I was curled up on one couch with a blanket, Ravi was in a chair, and Mom and Dad were sitting together across from us. Dad looked over at Mom and said, "Kids, we have some news we need to share." I laughed and said, almost jokingly, "What, do you have cancer or something?" And then they both looked at each other—and Dad said yes.

Everything after that felt surreal. I remember shock more than words. I could feel a part of me stepping out of the experience and observing myself—the rational side of my brain taking over and seeking information (so many questions), trying to understand what it meant, but ultimately all this falling to the wayside and the tears flowed. I remember wondering what was happening inside Ravi's head, because from the outside he just seemed very still. I don't remember what we talked about, or what we ate, or how the evening ended—only that feeling of disbelief and sadness hanging in the room.

The next day, when I was driving to pick up Vipul from BART and contemplating how I would share the news, I kept repeating to myself out loud—over and over—*keep moving forward, there is no other way*. It felt like that was the only option available at that moment. I told Vipul in the car, and when we came home, he gave Dad a big hug and didn't ask a lot of questions or make him repeat the diagnosis in painful detail. I really noticed that. He just tuned into what the family needed and quietly showed up. Throughout everything, he has been such a steadying force for me, and I remember thinking so many times how grateful I was to have such a loving partner while facing the possibility of losing Dad.

The diagnosis completely changed how I felt about our upcoming wedding. There was "Before," where we had what now feel like petty arguments about details—dresses, necklines, traditions, whether something felt "Indian enough." Then there was "After," where the wedding became about family and community and love. Watching Mom support Dad through those early days was so formative for me. It shaped how I understood marriage—being there for each other through the hard times—and that deeply influenced the vows I wrote.

One thing that was hard was that we all grieved differently. At first Dad didn't want to share the diagnosis widely, and while I respected that choice, my instinct was to reach out to friends, to cry with people I loved. There were also times when it felt like there wasn't much space to voice fear or sadness, because so much of Dad's approach centered on positivity and believing in healing. I understood why—and I supported it—but sometimes it meant that Mom and I carried a lot privately together.

I also carried a lot of worry for Mom. So much of my fear came from imagining her being alone. I kept thinking about her life ahead—how much time she still had, and what it would mean to live it without Dad. Back then, we didn't see each other as often as we do now, and it was harder for me to picture what life would look like if she came to live with us. I remember going on a walk with her in the early weeks of the diagnosis and she shared some of her fears for the future. My heart just shattered. It felt like there was nothing I could do to protect her from that suffering, and that helplessness was one of the hardest parts.

The chemo and radiation period was very tough, but I was so proud of Dad. He was uncomfortable and exhausted, losing weight, worn down—and still he moved through that time with so much grace and matter-of-fact acceptance. Mom had to make a trip to India for a few weeks during that time. Ravi, Vipul, and I took turns staying at home, working, and driving Dad to appointments. It was a strange period—heavy and tender at the same time—and I really saw him as a model for how to walk through something difficult with courage.

When Dad eventually decided not to continue with the standard treatments, that was incredibly hard for me to accept. Intellectually, I respected his independence—I knew it was his life and his choice—but emotionally, it brought up fear and also some anger. The doctors were saying he *should* do certain things, and I struggled to understand why he wouldn't fight for every possible chance to live longer. Over time, I've come to better understand his perspective—and I now believe much more in the path he chose, especially seeing how deeply healing and spirituality became part of his journey. But even now, years later, when Dad declines scans or treatments, I still feel that old fear surface. Becoming a parent has helped me better accept that his choices are his to make—even when they're hard for me to accept or understand.

By the time the bladder cancer diagnosis came, we were already so battle-hardened from everything before. It didn't land with the same shock, not because it wasn't serious, but because we were already living in this constant state of vigilance—bracing ourselves with every scan, every test result. It felt like *one more thing* layered onto an already exhausting emotional landscape. I think my body stayed in fight-or-flight mode for years.

And yet, through all of it, something transformational happened in our family. We stripped away so many unimportant frictions and learned to focus on what really matters: vulnerability, authenticity, acceptance, and showing up for each other in moments of crisis. Our bonds feel deeper now. We still argue, still have small conflicts—we're still a family—but the foundation underneath feels stronger.

In particular, I am inspired by how Mom has chosen to live her life in the face of Dad's diagnosis. She is building community through new friendships, finding nourishment through her love of nature and hiking, and experiencing newfound joy, love, and playfulness with her granddaughter. I worry far less now about how she would navigate life if Dad weren't here someday. I see her as someone who will not only survive, but live fully.

Looking back, I don't feel there's anything I wish we had done differently. There was pain, fear, and disagreement along the way, but those experiences shaped who we are now as a family. We say *I love you*—a lot. We stayed open. We stayed together. And because of that, I have no regrets.

A SON'S BATTLE ALONGSIDE HIS FATHER - RAVI'S PERSPECTIVE

The Call That Changed Everything

When Jaya and I were first going to be told about Dad's diagnosis, I remember Mom called us up on the phone. We had her on speaker, and I remember I had some work to do so I said I wasn't coming home.

Mom was a lot pushier than she normally would be. She kept saying, "Oh, you know, just don't worry about it. Just come home. Just come home this weekend."

I remember making a joke, something along the lines of, "I feel like you're going to tell us you have cancer or something." And she just said, "You guys should just come home."

Jaya and I looked at each other and talked on the way home about how weird it felt. So when Mom and Dad sat us down and told us it was in fact cancer, I remember thinking back to that joke I had made. It felt so surreal. I think I felt shell-shocked. I had a hard time knowing how to react. I couldn't really think about the future at that exact moment because I didn't know the details of how life would change.

Coming Home to Help

I have friends who have gone through cancer. I have lost friends to cancer. But even then, I think until you really have someone that you live with go through it and you see the small daily things they endure, it's hard to understand or imagine.

Over the following month or so, I came to terms with this idea that I had to be there—not only for Dad but also for Mom, who was going through her own mental trials and tribulations with all of this. I decided that I was going to quit my job and move back home to help.

I thought it would be a lot more practical help. I thought I'd be helping Dad do certain things because you hear about someone going through chemo and radiation—you hear about how much weaker they become. I didn't really have a clear understanding of what that meant or looked like. I didn't know if he was going to have trouble walking up the stairs. I didn't know what to expect. But in the end I think most of my support was being there for both of them emotionally, especially when tensions between them rose up.

Navigating Family Tensions

I think the secret struggle that comes with cancer is the impact it can have on relationships. I saw that with our Mom and Dad and how they would butt heads on all these extra things. Mom is such a caregiver that she wanted to do everything possible to really take care of our Dad and make sure he was getting the best care possible. So, when she disagreed with him about not wanting to go through standard treatment anymore, it really weighed on her. And I think it was tough on Dad as well.

I'm really amazed at how well Dad handled that extra stress and pressure, because I know it probably wasn't easy for him while he was going through everything else to also have so many of us—including myself— as naysayers to his approach, saying, "Please don't drop standard treatments. What are you doing?"

He really seemed to hold things together in this way that I really respect, because I think that must have been a mental struggle to be around that kind of negativity about his approach and to still hold true and fast against what all of these other people were saying. But he just trusted and believed that his body knew what was best for him, and he followed his gut on it.

And I mean, who can argue with the results? He's doing so well now. He outlived all the diagnoses and all of the expectations from doctors and all these people who really do know this stuff very well. I felt like I was at least able to help a little bit in being an extra set of ears for both Mom and Dad to vent to or talk through some of those trying times. And of course, being able to help logistically where I could.

The Feeling of Being at War

After Dad got that sentencing from the doctor of six months to live, suddenly every holiday, every event became really important. Every birthday wasn't an "oh yeah, we'll do something, maybe go out to dinner if we feel like it." It was "No, we're all going to be here for this dinner, for this birthday. We're all going to make sure we're home for Thanksgiving." Everything became urgent and precious.

One thing I don't really hear talked about by other families who go through cancer with a loved one is this switch that eventually flips in your head after maybe the first few weeks. It feels like you're at war. And it's strange because, outside of moving back home and trying to help out, I probably didn't actually have that much to do. Dad was the one doing the real battle. But it still felt like for our family, we were at war with this idea of cancer.

I remember talking with Jaya about this maybe half a year or a year in—there's just this feeling of combat that doesn't disengage after things start. It's a nonstop feeling that doesn't get turned off until enough time passes that things feel normal again.

A Moment of Peace

Jaya's wedding felt like a break from that constant vigilance. It was such a relief because it felt like we were able to be "off" for a little bit. We were able to just enjoy ourselves and be in that present moment and not be thinking about Dad having cancer or worrying about things. It was such a relief and such a joy to be around everyone in that free-hearted spirit.

That feeling does eventually start to fade off. But it took a while. Now, looking back on time, life feels very, very normal, especially with where all of the cancer stuff is these days. But it really did take years to progress mentally to not feel like there's an active combatant live on the scene.

Respecting His Path

Even now it's hard for me to gauge how dad was feeling during his treatments. He had this incredibly strong resolve to pursue his approach to the absolute fullest. He really believed in the way he was going to do things.

Maybe it's a testament to the kind of person he is. Through his business dealings as such a successful entrepreneur, Dad built into himself this identity that he doesn't need validation from everyone else to fully pursue and dive into what he believes is the solution or the right way to go. He's not someone who just follows trends. He makes the trend or he makes things happen.

I think you have to have a little of that attitude to go with the kind of approach that Dad went with and to come out the other end successfully.

Looking Back

I'm not sure if we could have done anything different. I feel like we did everything to the best of our capabilities with where we were. Sometimes, I do wonder at times if I could have been more helpful in other ways.

I wonder if Dad wasn't so strong-willed with the way he approached things, if he were someone else who didn't quite have that degree of confidence in his own approach, would we have been dissuading him and making it harder for him to continue that approach? That power of the mind to believe in the ability to heal yourself. Were we dampening that? I think about that sometimes.

But I think we did everything that we could with the people that we were at that time. I'm glad that we're much further along on all of this and that it feels very different now and much more manageable. I'm grateful for every day we get.

JOINING A FAMILY IN CRISIS: SON-IN-LAW'S PERSPECTIVE

The News Through Tears

I first heard about Dad's diagnosis on a Saturday when I took the BART from San Francisco to Fremont. Jaya came to pick me up, and even before she said anything, I could see something was very wrong. Her eyes were filled with tears, and the moment I got into the car, she broke down and shared the news. It was a shock. For the first fifteen seconds, it didn't register. There had been no sign that something this serious was happening—nothing about Dad's energy or health suggested this was coming.

Later that afternoon, at the Pareek home, Dad shared the news directly with me. At that point, I had only known him for about two years, maybe seen him twenty times. Even with that limited time, I felt a strong sense of sadness—both for what this meant for him personally and for what it meant for the family.

The prognosis that typically comes with GBM—six to nine months—is tough to wrap your head around. Jaya and I were only months away from our wedding, and I had been looking forward to getting to know Dad more deeply. Having spent fifteen years away from my own parents, I was looking forward to having another father figure in my life.

Memories of Cancer's Toll

My experience seeing an uncle go through cancer treatment shaped my reaction. His treatment had been incredibly difficult—physically transformative in ways that were hard to witness—and the process took a toll not just on him but on everyone around him. That memory made me worry about the suffering that might lie ahead for Dad, and for Mom, Jaya, and Ravi, who would be closest to it.

My mind also went to the structure of Jaya's family. I grew up in a large family in India: my parents, my two uncles, their families—sixteen of us who lived near each other and shared day-to-day life. When we went through grief, there was a wide network to absorb the emotional impact. In contrast, the Pareek family is small and private. I remember thinking how big the absence could feel if they lost Dad. I didn't fully know how to support Jaya in something like this—I only knew that the road ahead felt uncertain and heavy.

Coming to Terms with a Different Path

From the beginning, I sensed that Dad wasn't fully bought into standard treatment. Jaya mentioned privately that he was considering alternatives or had doubts about continuing with chemo, thinking more about quality of life. Initially, this caught me off guard because Dad had always struck me as a practical person, someone who evaluated odds, made decisions, and moved forward.

When he did begin chemo, there was collective relief—not necessarily because any of us were convinced it would be the answer, but because it felt like we were giving all options a fair attempt. But chemo was difficult for Dad. The energy in the Pareek home—usually light, humorous, centered around conversations and dinner—became more muted. Dad seemed quieter, understandably tired, and that shift affected the whole environment.

Around this time, I talked to a close friend whose mother had battled cancer for years. He shared that, looking back, he wished his family hadn't pursued every treatment available because the last years were extremely painful for her. That perspective helped me understand that Dad's hesitation wasn't about giving up; it might have been about wanting to live whatever time was left with dignity, comfort, and agency.

Over time, what helped me come to terms with his decision was recognizing that choices like this belong most to the person whose body and life are at the center of it. When I considered Dad's life—the responsibilities he carried, the generosity he showed to family members, supporting education for poor children, —it became clear that he had earned the right to choose the path that aligned with his values.

When Hope Met Another Blow

The bladder cancer diagnosis felt like a major setback just as it seemed like things were stabilizing. Dad had undergone successful surgery for GBM, a few months had passed, and there were no visible signs that pointed back to the original prognosis. There was a quiet sense building—even if unspoken—that maybe we were getting more time than expected.

When the second diagnosis came, it disrupted that growing hope. It felt like the family had just begun stitching together a new normal, and suddenly that was undone. The analogy that comes to mind is building something carefully—like a Jenga tower—only to have it collapse with one unexpected move. It wasn't dramatic; it was more like a quiet deflation, a reset back to uncertainty.

Celebration Amidst Crisis

Our wedding was in September, about five months after the original diagnosis. By that time, Dad had stopped chemo, had bladder cancer surgery behind him, and seemed more like himself again. The Pareek dinner table returned to its familiar rhythm—laughing, joking, and sharing wine.

Dad and Mom made a deliberate choice not to share details about his health widely. Even my own parents only knew that Dad had a tumor removed; they didn't know about the GBM diagnosis, the prognosis, or the second cancer. That helped create a space where the wedding could be celebrated as it was meant to be.

One detail that stands out is that Dad wore a hat to cover his scar. It resembled the style of Dev Anand, the famous Indian actor from the 60s. It became a talking point in a light-hearted way, instead of being a reminder of illness. In hindsight, that feels symbolic of how the family navigated that moment—choosing to emphasize joy, presence, and celebration rather than loss or fear.

Looking back, I think one of the most meaningful parts of that week was seeing Jaya fully present. In the months leading to the wedding, worry about Dad was always there in the background. The wedding created a rare pause from that weight. For me, it was surprising—in a good way—that amid such a difficult time, the family found room to celebrate deeply and genuinely.

The Power of Mindset

Six years into Dad's healing journey, it's hard not to reflect on how much has changed—not just in his health but in mindset across the family. It's possible that Dad is one of the fortunate cases who defied early expectations. At the same time, I've become more open to the idea that his approach—combining specific dietary choices, belief, and mindset—has influenced the trajectory of his journey.

One thing that stands out is how Dad's mindset reduced stress for everyone. His acceptance and positivity made the situation easier to talk about and easier to live with. There was less energy spent on fear or frustration, and more on living day-to-day life. That shift had practical benefits too—the family was able to function, stay connected, and maintain normal routines, instead of being consumed by worst-case thinking.

Some of Dad's ideas have influenced how I think about other parts of life. The idea of behaving as if you already are what you want to become—not just pretending, but genuinely feeling and carrying yourself that way—has been useful in work contexts. When I've approached projects or conversations as if I already belonged in the next phase of my career, I noticed that my decisions changed, my communication changed, and the way people responded also changed. Seeing Dad channel belief and intention into how he lives has made me more open to the idea that mindset isn't just abstract—it can shape behavior, which in turn can change results.

Looking back, we could have been more supportive sooner of Dad's decision not to continue standard treatment. But it's hard to know what to think in the moment. Our reactions came from wanting more time and from the examples we had seen. We didn't have many stories where alternative approaches were part of someone's healing, so the uncertainty felt risky and unfamiliar.

If we had known more stories like Dad's—examples of people prioritizing quality of life and mindset—we might have reached acceptance faster, with less emotional friction. But I don't fault anyone in the family for how they reacted at the time. We were trying to navigate something difficult with the information we had.

My hope is that this book finds its way not just to people considering similar approaches, but also to their families—the people who stand beside them and sometimes struggle with the decision differently. Understanding the reasoning doesn't remove the uncertainty, but it can make the journey feel less isolating and more shared.

As I read these words from my wife, children, and son-in-law, I am deeply moved by their courage, their love, and their transformation. Each of them fought their own battle—Anu with her spiritual awakening through surrender, Jaya with her journey from fear to acceptance, Ravi with his quiet strength as the family's emotional anchor, and Vipul with his evolution from uncertainty to understanding while navigating his new role in a family facing crisis. Their perspectives reveal the hidden struggles I couldn't fully see at the time: the weight of keeping secrets, the challenge of supporting my unconventional choices while harboring their own doubts, the constant state of "being at war" that they endured for years, and the delicate balance of joining a family while it faced its greatest challenge. Their journeys alongside mine have been equally challenging, perhaps more so in some ways, as they had to balance hope and fear, support and self-care, acceptance and advocacy. Their perspectives complete the picture of what healing truly means—not just for the patient, but for the entire family ecosystem that surrounds them with love.

EPILOGUE: THE JOURNEY CONTINUES

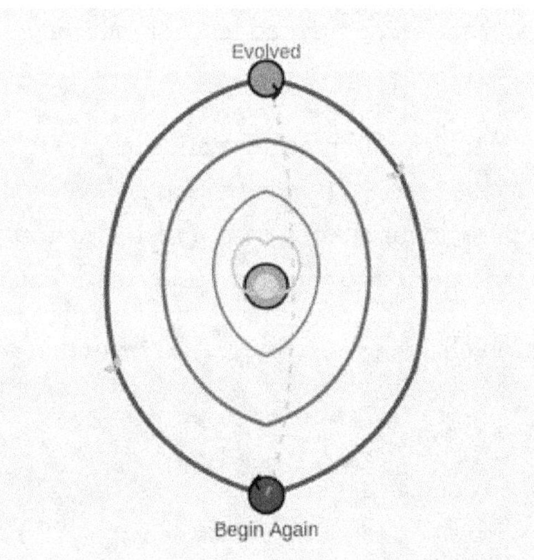

As I write this, 6 years have passed since my terminal diagnosis. The doctors who gave me months to live have watched in amazement as I've not just survived but thrived. Yet I want to be clear: this isn't a story about conquering cancer. It's about discovering that we are so much more than these bodies, and healing is so much more than physical recovery.

The MEDS Method remains my daily practice, but my relationship with it continues to evolve. Some days, I practice mechanically, simply going through the motions when I'm tired or distracted. Other days, each element becomes a doorway to transcendence. Both are perfect. The path accommodates us wherever we are. If you're facing a health crisis, or any major life challenge, know that you can start exactly where I did—desperate, mechanical, skeptical. You don't need to believe in consciousness or spirituality. You don't need to have faith. You just need to begin. Start with MEDS mechanically if that's all you can manage. But stay open. Through consistent practice, something deeper may emerge. You might discover, as I did, that healing the body is just the beginning of remembering who you really are.

This journey has no endpoint, only deepening. Each day brings new understanding, new dimensions of experience, new recognition of what we truly are. Cancer was my uninvited teacher, but the lessons it brought are universal.

The journey continues, and it begins with a single step: the willingness to see yourself not as broken, but as whole; not as a victim of circumstances, but as a participant in your own transformation; not as separate and alone, but as connected to the very source of life itself.

That recognition changes everything. And from that recognition, true healing begins.

∞

PART *Seven*

References and Resources

REFERENCES AND RESOURCES

A Comprehensive Guide for Your Healing Journey

This comprehensive reference guide includes all the books, articles, research studies, and resources that informed my healing journey and the creation of this book. These resources are organized by category to help you find the information most relevant to your specific needs and interests.

BOOKS

MEDITATION AND MIND-BODY HEALING

You Are the Placebo: Making Your Mind Matter by Dr. Joe Dispenza (Hay House, 2014)

Explores the science of how thoughts and beliefs can influence physical health and healing through documented case studies of spontaneous remissions.

Website: www.drjoedispenza.com

Becoming Supernatural: How Common People Are Doing the Uncommon by Dr. Joe Dispenza (Hay House, 2017)

Advanced techniques for meditation and transformation, with healing testimonials and scientific research on brain-wave patterns during meditation.

Breaking the Habit of Being Yourself: How to Lose Your Mind and Create a New One by Dr. Joe Dispenza (Hay House, 2012)

Details the neuroscience of change and epigenetics, providing practical meditation techniques for personal transformation.

You Can Heal Your Life by Louise L. Hay (Hay House, 1984)

The foundational text on affirmations and the mind-body connection. Has sold over 50 million copies worldwide and explores how thoughts create our physical reality.

Website: www.louisehay.com

Heal Your Body: The Mental Causes for Physical Illness by Louise L. Hay (Hay House, 1984)

A step-by-step guidebook listing ailments and their emotional causes, with corresponding healing affirmations.

The Power of Intention by Dr. Wayne W. Dyer (Hay House, 2004)

Explores intention as a force in the universe that allows creation to take place, explaining how to access this energy for healing and transformation.

Website: www.drwaynedyer.com

Wishes Fulfilled: Mastering the Art of Manifesting by Dr. Wayne W. Dyer (Hay House, 2012)

Combines spiritual wisdom with practical techniques for creating the life you desire through the power of the mind.

Excuses Begone!: How to Change Lifelong, Self-Defeating Thinking Habits by Dr. Wayne W. Dyer (Hay House, 2009)

Reveals how to change self-defeating thinking patterns that prevent living at the highest levels of success, happiness, and health.

There's a Spiritual Solution to Every Problem by Dr. Wayne W. Dyer (Hay House, 2001)

Demonstrates how moving to higher levels of spiritual consciousness can solve any problem.

Quantum Healing: Exploring the Frontiers of Mind/Body Medicine by Deepak Chopra, M.D. (Bantam Books, 1989)

Groundbreaking exploration of the mind-body connection using principles from quantum physics and Ayurvedic medicine.

Website: www.deepakchopra.com

The Healing Self: A Revolutionary New Plan to Supercharge Your Immunity by Deepak Chopra, M.D. & Rudolph E. Tanzi, Ph.D. (Harmony Books, 2018)

A comprehensive strategy to activate the body's healing system and engage the immune system in the healing response.

Perfect Health: The Complete Mind/Body Guide by Deepak Chopra, M.D. (Harmony Books, 1991)

The original guide to applying ancient Ayurvedic wisdom to everyday life, including identifying your mind-body type.

Total Meditation: Practices in Living the Awakened Life by Deepak Chopra, M.D. (Harmony Books, 2020)

A complete exploration of meditation's physical, mental, emotional, and spiritual benefits with a 52-week program.

The Relaxation Response by Herbert Benson, M.D. & Miriam Z. Klipper (HarperTorch, 2000)

The foundational text on the relaxation response and its physiological benefits for stress reduction and healing.

Full Catastrophe Living: Using the Wisdom of Your Body and Mind to Face Stress, Pain, and Illness by Jon Kabat-Zinn, Ph.D. (Bantam Books, 2013)

The definitive guide to Mindfulness-Based Stress Reduction (MBSR) from its founder, applicable to chronic illness and cancer.

Mindfulness-Based Cancer Recovery: A Step-by-Step MBSR Approach by Linda E. Carlson & Michael Speca (New Harbinger Publications, 2011)

A practical guide to mindfulness-based stress reduction specifically designed for cancer patients.

You Can Conquer Cancer: The Ground-Breaking Self-Help Classic by Ian Gawler (Michelle Anderson Publishing, 2013)

A comprehensive guide from a cancer survivor who pioneered mind-body approaches to cancer healing.

Love, Medicine and Miracles by Bernie S. Siegel, M.D. (William Morrow, 1998)

A surgeon's observations about the role of love, hope, and mind-body connection in exceptional cancer survivors.

Fighting Cancer From Within by Martin L. Rossman, M.D. (Holt Paperbacks, 2010)

Practical visualization and guided imagery techniques for cancer patients.

Cancer as a Turning Point by Lawrence LeShan, Ph.D. (Plume, 1989)

Explores the psychological and emotional dimensions of cancer and how addressing them can support healing.

NUTRITION AND DIET FOR CANCER HEALING

Eat to Beat Disease: The New Science of How Your Body Can Heal Itself by William W. Li, M.D. (Grand Central Publishing, 2019)

Explores how food activates the body's five defense systems, including anti-angiogenesis, to prevent and fight disease.

Website: www.drwilliamli.com

The Metabolic Approach to Cancer by Dr. Nasha Winters & Jess Higgins Kelley (Chelsea Green Publishing, 2017)

Written by a naturopathic oncologist who survived terminal cancer. Identifies 10 key terrain elements crucial to cancer management.

Keto for Cancer: Ketogenic Metabolic Therapy as a Targeted Nutritional Strategy by Miriam Kalamian (Chelsea Green Publishing, 2017)

Comprehensive guide to implementing ketogenic diet for cancer, with meal planning, recipes, and guidance for working with your medical team.

How to Starve Cancer by Jane McLelland (Agenor Publishing, 2018)

Terminal cancer survivor who developed a metabolic approach using a cancer-starving diet, supplements, and off-label drugs.

Tripping Over the Truth: How the Metabolic Theory of Cancer Is Overturning One of Medicine's Most Entrenched Paradigms by Travis Christofferson (Chelsea Green Publishing, 2014)

Explains how the metabolic theory of cancer is challenging conventional understanding, making complex science accessible.

Cancer as a Metabolic Disease by Thomas Seyfried, Ph.D. (Wiley, 2012)

The scientific foundation for the metabolic theory of cancer, showing cancer originates from damage to cellular respiration.

Foods to Fight Cancer by Richard Beliveau, Ph.D. & Denis Gingras, Ph.D. (DK Publishing, 2017)

Scientific research on anti-cancer foods and their mechanisms of action.

The Cancer-Fighting Kitchen by Rebecca Katz & Mat Edelson (Ten Speed Press, 2017)

Science-based recipes organized by symptoms and side effects, written by a culinary nutritionist specializing in cancer care.

Website: www.rebeccakatz.com

Chris Beat Cancer: A Comprehensive Plan for Healing Naturally by Chris Wark (Hay House, 2018)

Stage 3 colon cancer survivor who rejected chemotherapy after surgery and used evidence-based nutrition and natural therapies.

Website: www.chrisbeatcancer.com

Beat Cancer Kitchen: Deliciously Simple Plant-Based Anticancer Recipes by Chris Wark & Micah Wark (Hay House, 2021)

Companion cookbook with whole-food, plant-based recipes for healing and prevention.

The China Study by T. Colin Campbell, Ph.D. & Thomas M. Campbell (BenBella Books, 2016)

Landmark research on the relationship between diet and disease, including cancer.

The Gerson Therapy by Charlotte Gerson & Morton Walker (Kensington, 2006)

One of the first alternative cancer therapies with 60+ years of success, based on organic juicing, coffee enemas, and supplements.

Beating Cancer with Nutrition by Patrick Quillin, Ph.D. (Nutrition Times Press, 2005)

Author has 47 years experience including decade as VP of Nutrition at Cancer Treatment Centers of America.

How to Prevent and Treat Cancer with Natural Medicine by Michael T. Murray, N.D. (Riverhead Books, 2020)

Natural approaches to cancer prevention and treatment from a naturopathic doctor.

FUNCTIONAL MEDICINE AND LONGEVITY

Young Forever: The Secrets to Living Your Longest, Healthiest Life by Mark Hyman, M.D. (Little, Brown Spark, 2023)

Comprehensive guide to longevity and reversing biological aging through functional medicine approaches.

Website: www.drhyman.com

The Pegan Diet: 21 Practical Principles for Reclaiming Your Health by Mark Hyman, M.D. (Little, Brown Spark, 2021)

Combines the best aspects of paleo and vegan diets for optimal health.

Food Fix: How to Save Our Health, Our Economy, Our Communities, and Our Planet by Mark Hyman, M.D. (Little, Brown Spark, 2020)

Explores how our food system impacts health and provides solutions for transformation.

The Blood Sugar Solution by Mark Hyman, M.D. (Little, Brown Spark, 2012)

Reveals that balanced insulin levels are the secret to preventing diabetes, heart disease, cancer, and more.

Eat Fat, Get Thin by Mark Hyman, M.D. (Little, Brown Spark, 2016)

Why the fat we eat is the key to sustained weight loss and vibrant health.

SPIRITUALITY AND EMOTIONAL HEALING

Dying to Be Me: My Journey from Cancer, to Near Death, to True Healing by Anita Moorjani (Hay House, 2012)

> *After Stage 4 Hodgkin's lymphoma caused her organs to shut down, the author had a near-death experience and recovered completely within weeks.*

> Website: www.anitamoorjani.com

Radical Remission: Surviving Cancer Against All Odds by Kelly A. Turner, Ph.D. (HarperOne, 2014)

> *Research on over 1,000 cases of radical remission. Identifies 9 key healing factors common among survivors.*

> Website: www.radicalremission.com

Radical Hope: 10 Key Healing Factors from Exceptional Survivors by Kelly A. Turner, Ph.D. & Tracy White (Hay House, 2020)

> *Follow-up with updated research, adding 'Exercise' as the 10th healing factor.*

The Power of Now: A Guide to Spiritual Enlightenment by Eckhart Tolle (New World Library, 1997)

> *A spiritual classic on presence and consciousness that has helped millions find inner peace.*

When Things Fall Apart: Heart Advice for Difficult Times by Pema Chodron (Shambhala, 1997)

> *Buddhist wisdom for navigating life's challenges with courage and compassion.*

Kitchen Table Wisdom: Stories That Heal by Rachel Naomi Remen, M.D. (Riverhead Books, 2006)

> *Healing stories from a physician who has worked with cancer patients for decades.*

Close to the Bone: Life-Threatening Illness as a Soul Journey by Jean Shinoda Bolen, M.D. (Conari Press, 2007)

> *Explores illness as a transformative spiritual journey.*

The Healing Journey: Overcoming the Crisis of Cancer by Alastair J. Cunningham, Ph.D. (Key Porter Books, 2012)

A psychologist's guide to the emotional and spiritual dimensions of cancer healing.

INTEGRATIVE AND HOLISTIC APPROACHES

Integrative Oncology by Donald Abrams, M.D. & Andrew Weil, M.D. (Oxford University Press, 2014)

The definitive medical textbook on integrative approaches to cancer care from leading experts at UCSF and University of Arizona.

Anticancer: A New Way of Life by David Servan-Schreiber, M.D., Ph.D. (Viking, 2009)

A neuroscientist and brain cancer survivor's integrative approach. Emphasizes anti-inflammatory diet, stress reduction, exercise, and environmental factors. Author lived 20 years after brain cancer diagnosis.

Anticancer Living: Transform Your Life and Health with the Mix of Six by Lorenzo Cohen, Ph.D. & Alison Jefferies (Viking, 2018)

The 'Mix of Six' lifestyle factors for cancer prevention and healing from MD Anderson Cancer Center research.

Natural Health, Natural Medicine by Andrew Weil, M.D. (Houghton Mifflin, 2004)

Comprehensive natural health guide from a pioneer in integrative medicine.

Website: www.drweil.com

Spontaneous Healing by Andrew Weil, M.D. (Ballantine Books, 1995)

How to discover and embrace your body's natural ability to maintain and heal itself.

The Truth About Cancer by Ty M. Bollinger (Hay House, 2017)

After losing 7 family members to cancer, author researched alternative treatments worldwide.

Outside the Box Cancer Therapies by Mark Stengler, N.D. & Paul Anderson, N.D. (Hay House, 2019)

Overview of alternative and complementary cancer therapies from naturopathic doctors.

The Definitive Guide to Cancer by Lise N. Alschuler, N.D. & Karolyn A. Gazella (Celestial Arts, 2013)

Comprehensive guide to integrative cancer treatment including supplements.

Life Over Cancer by Keith I. Block, M.D. (Bantam Books, 2009)

Comprehensive integrative cancer treatment program from the Block Center for Integrative Cancer Treatment.

Choices in Healing: Integrating the Best of Conventional and Complementary Approaches by Michael Lerner, Ph.D. (MIT Press, 1996)

Thoughtful guide to navigating treatment choices from the founder of Commonweal Cancer Help Program.

Michael A. Singer

Website: untetheredsoul.com

#1 New York Times bestselling author and founder of Temple of the Universe meditation center. Featured on Oprah's Super Soul Sunday. His works offer profound insights on consciousness, letting go, and inner freedom.

Living Untethered: Beyond the Human Predicament by Michael A. Singer (New Harbinger, 2022)

The Surrender Experiment: My Journey into Life's Perfection by Michael A. Singer (Harmony, 2015)

The Untethered Soul: The Journey Beyond Yourself by Michael A. Singer (New Harbinger, 2007)

David R. Hawkins, M.D., Ph.D.

Website: veritaspub.com (Official Publisher)

Psychiatrist, physician, and internationally renowned consciousness researcher (1927-2012). Developed the Map of Consciousness calibration system. Co-authored work with Nobel Laureate Linus Pauling. Received praise from Mother Teresa for his writings.

Transcending the Levels of Consciousness: The Stairway to Enlightenment by David R. Hawkins, M.D., Ph.D. (Hay House, 2006)

Letting Go: The Pathway of Surrender by David R. Hawkins, M.D., Ph.D. (Hay House, 2012)

Power vs. Force: The Hidden Determinants of Human Behavior by David R. Hawkins, M.D., Ph.D. (Hay House, 1995)

Bruce H. Lipton, Ph.D.

Website: www.brucelipton.com

Cell biologist and recipient of the 2009 Goi Peace Award. Former medical school professor at University of Wisconsin and Stanford researcher. Pioneer in understanding how beliefs and environment influence gene expression (epigenetics).

Spontaneous Evolution: Our Positive Future and a Way to Get There by Bruce H. Lipton, Ph.D. & Steve Bhaerman (Hay House, 2009)

The Honeymoon Effect: The Science of Creating Heaven on Earth by Bruce H. Lipton, Ph.D. (Hay House, 2013)

The Biology of Belief: Unleashing the Power of Consciousness, Matter & Miracles by Bruce H. Lipton, Ph.D. (Hay House, 2005)

Gregg Braden

Website: greggbraden.com

Five-time New York Times bestselling author and pioneer bridging science, spirituality, and human potential. Former computer systems designer for Cisco and Fortune 500 companies. His work explores how beliefs shape biology and reality.

Pure Human: The Hidden Truth of Our Divinity, Power, and Destiny by Gregg Braden (Hay House, 2024)

The Spontaneous Healing of Belief: Shattering the Paradigm of False Limits by Gregg Braden (Hay House, 2008)

The Divine Matrix: Bridging Time, Space, Miracles, and Belief by Gregg Braden (Hay House, 2007)

Andrew Huberman, Ph.D.

Website: www.hubermanlab.com

Stanford neuroscientist and host of the #1 health podcast Huberman Lab. Discusses science-based tools for sleep, stress, focus, and performance. Features episodes on meditation, breathwork, and mind-body practices.

Protocols: An Operating Manual for the Human Body by Andrew Huberman, Ph.D. (Upcoming)

SCIENTIFIC RESEARCH AND MEDICAL LITERATURE

MEDITATION AND MIND-BODY RESEARCH

QUANTUM Study (QUest to ANalyze a Thousand hUmans Meditating)

Led by Dr. Hemal H. Patel, Ph.D., Professor and Vice Chair for Research, Department of Anesthesiology, UC San Diego School of Medicine. This groundbreaking study assesses the impact of meditation on nearly 2,000 individuals undergoing intensive meditative experiences, examining physiological, biochemical, and molecular changes. Funded by a $10 million commitment from Inner-Science Research Fund.

Contact: https://today.ucsd.edu/story/10m-from-innerscience-research-fund-will-fuel-study-on-meditation-to-combat-disease

Key Research Papers

Ornish, D., et al. (2008). Changes in prostate gene expression in men undergoing an intensive nutrition and lifestyle intervention. Proceedings of the National Academy of Sciences, 105(24), 8369-8374.

Cole, S.W. (2019). The conserved transcriptional response to adversity. Current Opinion in Behavioral Sciences, 28, 31-37.

Epel, E.S., et al. (2004). Accelerated telomere shortening in response to life stress. Proceedings of the National Academy of Sciences, 101(49), 17312-17315.

Kiecolt-Glaser, J.K., et al. (2010). Stress, inflammation, and yoga practice. Psychosomatic Medicine, 72(2), 113-121.

Lutgendorf, S.K. & Sood, A.K. (2011). Biobehavioral factors and cancer progression. Psychosomatic Medicine, 73(9), 724-730.

NUTRITION AND CANCER RESEARCH

Aggarwal, B.B. & Sung, B. (2009). Pharmacological basis for the role of curcumin in chronic diseases: An age-old spice with modern targets. Trends in Pharmacological Sciences, 30(2), 85-94.

Farvid, M.S., et al. (2021). Consumption of sugar-sweetened beverages and cancer risk. Critical Reviews in Food Science and Nutrition, 61(13), 2255-2273.

Lauby-Secretan, B., et al. (2016). Body fatness and cancer—viewpoint of the IARC Working Group. New England Journal of Medicine, 375(8), 794-798.

SLEEP AND IMMUNITY RESEARCH

Irwin, M.R. (2019). Sleep and inflammation: Partners in sickness and in health. Nature Reviews Immunology, 19(11), 702-715.

Booth, F.W., Roberts, C.K., & Laye, M.J. (2012). Lack of exercise is a major cause of chronic diseases. Comprehensive Physiology, 2(2), 1143-1211.

MAJOR MEDICAL CENTER RESOURCES

UCSF OSHER CENTER FOR INTEGRATIVE HEALTH

The UCSF Osher Center for Integrative Health offers comprehensive integrative cancer care, combining conventional medicine with evidence-based complementary therapies. Led by experts including Dr. Donald Abrams, a world-renowned integrative oncologist.

Integrative Cancer Care Program
Individual consultations with integrative medicine providers specializing in cancer care, oncology group visits, and classes on nutrition, botanical therapies, and mind-body practices.

https://osher.ucsf.edu/patient-care/clinical-specialties/integrative-cancer-care

Dr. Donald Abrams' Video Series on Integrative Cancer Care
Four-part video series covering cancer nutrition, plant therapies, and non-traditional medicine for cancer patients.

https://osher.ucsf.edu/resources/dr-donald-abrams-four-part-video-series-integrative-cancer-care

Cancer and Nutrition Resource Guide
Evidence-based nutrition guidelines for cancer prevention and survivorship.

https://osher.ucsf.edu/patient-care/integrative-medicine-resources/cancer-and-nutrition

MAYO CLINIC INTEGRATIVE ONCOLOGY

Mayo Clinic's integrative oncology program combines Western medicine with evidence-based complementary therapy, so treatments are researched and proven to be effective.

Integrative Oncology Program

Comprehensive integrative cancer care including nutrition counseling, mind-body practices, acupuncture, massage therapy, and lifestyle medicine.

https://www.mayoclinic.org/departments-centers/integrative-oncology/overview/ovc-20542190

Cancer Education Center

Free virtual classes exploring integrative medicine practices for cancer patients.

https://cancerblog.mayoclinic.org

Complementary and Alternative Medicine

Information on various integrative approaches including acupuncture, massage, meditation, and more.

https://www.mayoclinic.org/tests-procedures/complementary-alternative-medicine/about/pac-20393581

DUKE INTEGRATIVE MEDICINE

Duke Integrative Medicine Center offers customized, patient-centered health care that combines conventional medicine with proven complementary treatments, including specialized programs for cancer patients.

Duke Integrative Medicine Center

Full-service integrative primary care, programs, and workshops for whole-person healing.

https://dukeintegrativemedicine.org

Mindful Yoga for Cancer Program

Specialized yoga therapy program designed for cancer patients and survivors.

https://dhwprograms.dukehealth.org/programs-training/

Mindfulness-Based Stress Reduction (MBSR)

Evidence-based mindfulness program for stress reduction and emotional well-being.

https://dhwprograms.dukehealth.org

MEMORIAL SLOAN KETTERING INTEGRATIVE MEDICINE

Integrative Medicine Service

Comprehensive integrative therapies including acupuncture, massage, music therapy, and mind-body practices for cancer patients.

https://www.mskcc.org/cancer-care/diagnosis-treatment/
symptom-management/integrative-medicine

About Herbs Database

Evidence-based information on herbs, botanicals, supplements, and more for cancer patients.

https://www.mskcc.org/cancer-care/integrative-medicine/herbs

MD ANDERSON CANCER CENTER

Integrative Medicine Center

Comprehensive integrative oncology services including acupuncture, meditation, nutrition counseling, and oncology massage.

https://www.mdanderson.org/patients-family/
diagnosis-treatment/care-centers-clinics/
integrative-medicine-center.html

NATIONAL CANCER INSTITUTE (NCI)

Complementary and Alternative Medicine (CAM)

Comprehensive information on CAM therapies used in cancer care, current research, and how to evaluate treatments.

https://www.cancer.gov/about-cancer/treatment/cam

YOUTUBE CHANNELS AND VIDEO RESOURCES

MIND-BODY AND MEDITATION

Dr. Joe Dispenza

Transformative meditations, healing testimonials, and lectures on the science of changing your mind to heal your body.

https://www.youtube.com/@DrJoeDispenza

Hay House

Official channel featuring Louise Hay, Wayne Dyer, Deepak Chopra, and other transformational teachers.

https://www.youtube.com/@hayhouse

Deepak Chopra

Meditations, wellness advice, and discussions on consciousness and healing.

https://www.youtube.com/@DeepakChopra

The Chopra Well

Guided meditations, wellness tips, and spiritual teachings.

https://www.youtube.com/@thechoprawell

https://www.youtube.com/@hubaboratory

Science-based protocols for sleep, stress, focus, and optimal performance from Stanford neuroscientist.

Huberman Lab

https://www.youtube.com/@GreggBradenOfficial

Science and spirituality lectures on human potential, consciousness, and healing.

Gregg Braden

https://www.youtube.com/@brucelipton

Lectures on epigenetics, the biology of belief, and how thoughts affect cells.

Bruce Lipton

https://www.youtube.com/@michaelsingerpodcast

Teachings on consciousness, meditation, and inner freedom from The Untethered Soul author.

Michael Singer

NUTRITION AND NATURAL HEALING

Chris Beat Cancer

Interviews with cancer survivors, nutrition information, and natural healing strategies.

https://www.youtube.com/@chrisbeatcancer

Dr. Mark Hyman

Functional medicine insights, nutrition advice, and health transformation strategies.

https://www.youtube.com/@MarkHymanMD

NutritionFacts.org

Evidence-based nutrition information with Dr. Michael Greger.

https://www.youtube.com/@NutritionFactsOrg

Dr. William Li

How food activates the body's defense systems and fights disease.

https://www.youtube.com/@DrWilliamLi

INTEGRATIVE ONCOLOGY

UCSF Osher Center

Educational videos on integrative approaches to cancer care.

https://www.youtube.com/@UCSFOsherCenter

The Truth About Cancer

Documentary series and interviews on alternative cancer treatments.

https://www.youtube.com/@tabornevideos

Radical Remission Project

Stories of radical remission and the 10 healing factors from Kelly Turner's research.

https://www.youtube.com/@radicalremission

PODCASTS

CANCER AND HEALING

Chris Beat Cancer Podcast
Interviews with cancer survivors using natural methods and integrative approaches.
https://www.chrisbeatcancer.com/podcast

The Radical Remission Podcast
Kelly Turner, Ph.D. interviews exceptional survivors and explores the 10 healing factors.

https://radicalremission.com/podcast

Cancer Secrets Podcast
Dr. Jonathan Stegall discusses integrative oncology approaches.

https://cancersecretsbook.com/podcast

Outside the Box Cancer Therapies Podcast
Dr. Mark Stengler explores integrative cancer treatments.

https://outsidetheboxcancertherapies.com

FUNCTIONAL MEDICINE AND WELLNESS

The Doctor's Farmacy with Dr. Mark Hyman
Conversations with leading experts on functional medicine, nutrition, and health transformation.

https://drhyman.com/podcast

The Model Health Show with Shawn Stevenson

Science-based nutrition, sleep, and wellness information.

https://themodelhealthshow.com

The Rich Roll Podcast

Plant-based nutrition and wellness transformation stories.

https://www.richroll.com/podcast

Feel Better, Live More with Dr. Rangan Chatterjee

Practical health and wellness advice from a UK physician.

https://drchatterjee.com/podcast

MIND-BODY AND SPIRITUALITY

Hay House Meditations

Guided meditations from Hay House authors including Dr. Joe Dispenza, Wayne Dyer, and more.
https://open.spotify.com/show/4zC7ylMB0iFYyv1p19yS7g

On Purpose with Jay Shetty

Conversations on mindfulness, purpose, and personal growth.
https://jayshetty.me/podcast

The Daily Meditation Podcast

Daily guided meditations for stress relief and healing.

https://www.thedailymeditationpodcast.com

https://www.hubermanlab.com/podcast

#1 health podcast discussing neuroscience, sleep, stress, meditation, and science-based wellness tools.

Huberman Lab Podcast

https://untetheredsoul.com/podcast

Deep teachings on consciousness, surrender, and inner freedom with Sounds True.

The Michael Singer Podcast

WEBSITES AND ONLINE RESOURCES

MIND-BODY AND MEDITATION RESOURCES

Dr. Joe Dispenza Official Website

Meditations, events, online courses, and scientific research on transformation and healing.

https://drjoedispenza.com

Dr. Wayne Dyer Official Website

Books, audio programs, and teachings on intention and spiritual growth.

https://www.drwaynedyer.com

Deepak Chopra Official Website

Wellness resources, meditations, and programs on mind-body health.

https://www.deepakchopra.com

UCLA Mindful Awareness Research Center

Free guided meditations and mindfulness resources.

https://www.uclahealth.org/uclamindful

Mindfulness-Based Cancer Recovery

Resources and information on MBSR specifically for cancer patients.

https://www.mindfulcancerrecovery.com

INTEGRATIVE CANCER ORGANIZATIONS

Society for Integrative Oncology

Professional organization advancing evidence-based integrative oncology.

https://integrativeonc.org

The Radical Remission Project

Research, resources, and community for radical remission survivors.

https://radicalremission.com

Anticancer Living

Resources based on the 'Mix of Six' lifestyle factors from MD Anderson research.

https://anticancerliving.com

Block Center for Integrative Cancer Treatment

Comprehensive integrative cancer care center.

https://www.blockmd.com

CommonWeal Cancer Help Program

Residential retreat programs for people with cancer.

https://www.commonweal.org/cancer-help

Healing Strong

Community-based support groups using biblical and nutritional approaches.

https://healingstrong.org

NUTRITION AND DIET RESOURCES

NutritionFacts.org

Evidence-based nutrition information and research summaries.

https://nutritionfacts.org

Chris Beat Cancer

Nutrition protocols, survivor interviews, and healing resources.

https://www.chrisbeatcancer.com

American Institute for Cancer Research

Research-based information on diet and cancer prevention.

https://www.aicr.org

Dr. William Li - Eat to Beat Disease

Resources on using food to activate the body's defense systems.

https://www.drwilliamli.com

RESEARCH AND CLINICAL TRIALS

ClinicalTrials.gov

Database of clinical trials including integrative cancer studies.

https://clinicaltrials.gov

PubMed

Database of medical research literature.

https://pubmed.ncbi.nlm.nih.gov

National Center for Complementary and Integrative Health (NCCIH)

NIH resource for research on complementary health approaches.

https://www.nccih.nih.gov

PATIENT SUPPORT COMMUNITIES

Cancer Support Community

Free emotional and social support for people affected by cancer.

https://www.cancersupportcommunity.org

CancerCare

Free professional support services including counseling and support groups.

https://www.cancercare.org

Cancer Hope Network

One-on-one peer support matching cancer patients with survivors.

https://www.cancerhopenetwork.org

CaringBridge

Personal health journey websites to connect with friends and family.

https://www.caringbridge.org

MOBILE APPS

MEDITATION AND MINDFULNESS

Insight Timer

Free meditation library with cancer support groups and thousands of guided meditations.

https://insighttimer.com

Headspace

Meditation app with cancer-specific programs for patients and caregivers.

https://www.headspace.com

Calm

Sleep stories, meditation, and anxiety reduction programs.

https://www.calm.com

Ten Percent Happier

Meditation and mindfulness practices with expert teachers.

https://www.tenpercent.com

Waking Up (Sam Harris)

Meditation app focusing on consciousness and well-being.

https://www.wakingup.com

Hay House Unlimited Audio

Unlimited access to Hay House audiobooks, meditations, and lectures.

https://www.empoweryouaudio.com

NUTRITION AND HEALTH TRACKING

Cronometer

Detailed nutrition and micronutrient tracking.

https://cronometer.com

MyFitnessPal

Nutrition tracking and meal planning.

https://www.myfitnesspal.com

SLEEP AND RECOVERY

Sleep Cycle

Sleep quality tracking and smart alarm.

https://www.sleepcycle.com

DOCUMENTARY FILMS

Heal (2017)

Directed by Kelly Noonan Gores. Explores the mind-body connection and our ability to heal ourselves, featuring Deepak Chopra, Bruce Lipton, and others.

https://www.healwithkelly.co

The C Word (2016)

Directed by Meghan O'Hara. Morgan Freeman narrates this exploration of cancer prevention and treatment strategies.

https://thecwordmovie.com

The Truth About Cancer: A Global Quest (2015)

Ty Bollinger's documentary series exploring alternative cancer treatments around the world.

https://thetruthaboutcancer.com

Forks Over Knives (2011)

Directed by Lee Fulkerson. Examines how a plant-based diet can prevent and reverse disease.

https://www.forksoverknives.com

What the Health (2017)

Directed by Kip Andersen. Explores the connection between diet and disease.

https://www.whatthehealthfilm.com

The Game Changers (2018)

Directed by Louie Psihoyos. Explores plant-based nutrition and athletic performance.

https://gamechangersmovie.com

Fantastic Fungi (2019)

Directed by Louie Schwartzberg. Explores the magical world of fungi and their medicinal properties.

https://fantasticfungi.com

A NOTE ON USING THESE RESOURCES

Remember that every healing journey is unique. What works for one person may not work for another. Use these resources as a starting point for your own research and always consult with qualified healthcare professionals before making significant changes to your treatment plan.

The inclusion of a resource in this list does not constitute an endorsement of all its content or claims. I encourage you to approach all information with both an open mind and healthy skepticism, taking what resonates with you and leaving what doesn't.

Most importantly, trust your intuition. You know your body better than anyone else. Let these resources inform and empower you, but always listen to your inner wisdom when making decisions about your health and healing.

www.ingramcontent.com/pod-product-compliance
Lightning Source LLC
Chambersburg PA
CBHW071430130726
47997CB00006B/2030